全面了解针灸在全球范围内的标准化进程、
循证实践的现状以及未来的前景

Acupuncture Standardization and Evidence-based Practice

针灸标准化与循证实践

主审 石学敏 王燕平
主编 史楠楠 梁宁
副主编 晏利姣 李慧珍 张海力

中医古籍出版社
Publishing House of Ancient Chinese Medical Books

中国中医药循证医学中心
China Center for Evidence Based Traditional Chinese Medicine

中国中医科学院中医临床基础医学研究所
Institute of Basic Research in Clinical Medicine, China Academy of Chinese Medical Sciences

图书在版编目（CIP）数据

针灸标准化与循证实践 / 史楠楠，梁宁主编. 北京 ：中医古籍出版社，2024. 8. -- ISBN 978-7-5152-2867-9

Ⅰ. R245

中国国家版本馆 CIP 数据核字第 2024RK0594 号

针灸标准化与循证实践

主编　史楠楠　梁　宁

出 版 人　李　淳
责任编辑　吴　頔
封面设计　王　磊
出版发行　中医古籍出版社
社　　址　北京市东城区东直门内南小街 16 号（100700）
电　　话　010-64089446（总编室）010-64002949（发行部）
网　　址　www.zhongyiguji.com.cn
印　　刷　北京中献拓方科技发展有限公司
开　　本　787mm×1092mm　1/16
印　　张　8.5
字　　数　179 千字
版　　次　2024 年 8 月第 1 版　2024 年 8 月第 1 次印刷
书　　号　ISBN 978-7-5152-2867-9
定　　价　58.00 元

Standardization
Evidence-based Practice

全面了解针灸在全球范围内的标准化进程
循证实践的现状以及未来的前景

《针灸标准化与循证实践》编辑委员会

主　审

石学敏　王燕平

主　编

史楠楠　梁　宁

副主编

晏利姣　李慧珍　张海力

编　委

（按照姓氏笔画排序）

王丁熠　车前子　田紫煜
刘　斌　李衣芗　张钰菁
张雪飞　陈　昭　林甲昊
宗星煜　赵国桢　胡紫腾
郭　敬　龚照元

序言

中医药作为我国传统医学的瑰宝，深植于千年文化沉淀之中，却在现代医学发展的浪潮中也面临着一些不容忽视的挑战。传统医学以经验和传统知识为基础，缺乏系统的标准和科学的验证和评估体系，这导致了一些问题的存在，例如治疗效果难以量化和评估、医疗实践的差异性较大、治疗手法缺乏规范等。为了更好地适应当代医学的要求，中医药迫切需要标准和循证医学的引入，以提高其可信性、可行性和临床应用的规范性。

标准，是我们认知事物的准则，是学科成熟程度的标志，更是中医药学科发展不可或缺的支持。近年来，中医药标准化工作有了更好、更快、更大的发展，形成了中医药专家广泛参与，全行业关注、支持和参与标准化建设的良好氛围，中医药标准制修订步伐明显加快，相对独立、完整的中医药标准体系框架初步形成。中医药标准化工作的支撑体系建设得到进一步加强，涌现出一批能够承担中医药标准化研究制定的组织机构，凝聚起一支医教研产相互配合、精通中医专业技术、熟悉标准管理知识的复合型专家队伍。国际标准化工作取得了突破性进展，我国实质性参与了世界卫生组织（WHO）国际疾病分类第十一次修订本（ICD-11）传统医学部分的制定，在国际标准化组织中医药技术委员会（ISO/TC249）平台，截至2024 年 7 月中方已发布中医药国际标准 73 项，在研中医药国际标准 22 项，4 名中方专家担任国际工作组召集人席位，这是具有跨时代意义的重大成就。中医临床实践指南作为规范中医医疗行为的一种特殊“标准”类型，近些年也取得了惊人的发展。2007 年，在 WHO 西太区的资助下，中国中医科学院组织编写了国内第一批中医循证临床实践指南。截至 2020 年 12 月，我国已经制定了 245 部指南 / 共识，涵盖了内、外、妇、儿等各科临床常见病，并在全国范围内推广应用。

20 世纪末，循证医学崭露头角，崛起为指导全球医疗活动的主流方法，临床研究证据逐渐替代医生临床经验，成为医疗活动应用决策的主要依据。这一方法不仅改变了医学思维的方式，也深刻影响了医学不同领域的发展。循证医学方法学为中医药学发展注入新的活力，为中医临床医疗决策标准化和中医药临床疗效做出客观、可信、系统的评价。应用循证医学的方法开展中医药学临床疗效评价，可以帮助我们寻找有效的中医药临床治疗的药物、方法、技术、措施等，进一步优化中医药资源配置与利用。

针灸，作为中医药学的重要组成部分，通过标准化和循证医学的推动，为整个中医药学科的发展提供了成功的案例。《针灸标准化与循证实践》一书以标准化和循证医学为主题，深入剖析了针灸疗法的现状和未来发展。我们不仅能够更深入地理解这一古老疗法的本质，也能够为其在当代医学中的应用提供更为明确的方向。这是一次有益的尝试，旨在推动传统医学与现代医学的交融，为中医药学科的创新注入新的动力，为医学研究提供更为全面深入的视角。透过本书，您将全面了解针灸在全球范围内的标准化进程、循证实践的现状以及未来的前景。

祝愿您在阅读的过程中获得充实的收获与启迪。

Preface

Traditional Chinese Medicine (TCM), a treasured heritage of our nation's traditional medical practice, is deeply rooted in millennia of cultural accumulation. However, it faces some undeniable challenges amidst the surge of modern medical developments. Traditional medicine, based on experience and traditional knowledge, lacks a systematic standard and scientific verification and evaluation system. This results in several issues, such as difficulties in quantifying and evaluating therapeutic effects, significant variations in medical practice, and a lack of standardized treatment methods. To better adapt to the demands of contemporary medicine, TCM urgently needs the introduction of standards and evidence-based medicine to enhance its credibility, feasibility, and clinical application norms.

Standards are the criteria by which we understand things, a mark of a discipline's maturity, and an indispensable support for the development of TCM. In recent years, the standardization of TCM has seen better, faster, and greater progress, creating an atmosphere where TCM experts widely participate, and the entire industry focuses on and supports standardization efforts. The pace of TCM standard formulation and revision has significantly accelerated, and a relatively independent and complete TCM standard system framework has initially formed. The support system for TCM standardization work has been further strengthened, leading to the emergence of organizations capable of undertaking TCM standardization research and formulation. A team of composite experts proficient in TCM professional technology and familiar with standard management knowledge has been assembled, and significant breakthroughs have been made in international standardization work. Our country has substantively participated in the formulation of the traditional medicine part of the World Health Organization's (WHO) International Classification of Diseases (ICD-11). On the platform of the International Organization for Standardization's TCM Technical Committee (ISO/TC249), as of July 2024 China has released 73 international standards for TCM and is currently working on 22 additional ones, with four Chinese experts serving as conveners of international working groups—an epoch-making achievement. As a special type of "standard" to regulate TCM medical practices, TCM clinical practice guidelines have also seen remarkable development in recent years. In 2007, with funding from the WHO Western Pacific Region, the China Academy of Chinese Medical Sciences organized the development of the first batch of evidence-based clinical practice guidelines for traditional Chinese medicine in China. As of December 2020, China has established 245 guidelines/consensuses covering common clinical diseases in internal medicine, surgery, gynecology, pediatrics, and other specialties, which have been widely promoted and applied nationwide.

At the end of the 20th century, evidence-based medicine emerged as the mainstream method guiding global medical activities. Clinical research evidence gradually replaced clinical experience as the main basis for medical decision-making. This approach not only changed the way we think about medicine but also profoundly influenced the development of various medical fields. Evidence-based medicine methodology has injected new vitality into TCM development, providing an objective and credible systematic evaluation of TCM clinical efficacy and standardizing TCM clinical decision-making. Applying evidence-based medicine methods to evaluate TCM clinical efficacy can help us identify effective TCM clinical treatments, methods, techniques, and measures, further optimizing the allocation and utilization of TCM resources.

Acupuncture, an important component of TCM, provides a successful case through the promotion of standardization and evidence-based medicine, contributing to the overall development of the TCM discipline. The book "Standardization and Evidence-Based Practice of Acupuncture" focuses on standardization and evidence-based medicine, delving deeply into the current status and future development of acupuncture therapy. This book not only allows us to understand the essence of this ancient therapy more deeply but also provides a clearer direction for its application in modern medicine. This is a beneficial attempt to promote the integration of traditional and modern medicine, injecting new impetus into the innovation of TCM and providing a more comprehensive and in-depth perspective for medical research. Through this book, you will gain a comprehensive understanding of the standardization process of acupuncture worldwide, the current state of evidence-based practice, and future prospects.

I wish you fruitful gains and inspiration during your reading.

Xuemin Shi

前言

在现代医学实践中，标准化和循证医学是确保医疗质量、推动医学进步的两个关键支柱。标准化提供了通用的技术语言，使不同地区、不同文化的医学实践可以在同一标准下进行对话与合作。而循证医学则通过系统性的研究与验证，确保医疗决策基于最新、最可靠的科学证据。针灸疗法作为一项历史悠久且应用广泛的中医传统治疗手段，已经在标准化和循证医学研究方面取得了显著进展。这种结合传统智慧与现代科学的方式，使得针灸逐渐融入全球医学实践，并在不同文化和社会背景中展现其独特的价值，为患者提供了更安全、更可靠的治疗选择。

本书共分为三个部分。第一部分将带领您穿越千年岁月，深入了解针灸在不同文明和时代的演变，并重点介绍针灸文明发展史上的重要医学经典著作，包括《黄帝内经》《灵枢》《难经》《针灸甲乙经》等。我们追溯其源流，探讨其传播与发展，从立法、教育、国际交流等方面系统梳理了针灸在当代全球化背景下，如何成为跨越国界的疗法并取得瞩目成就。截至目前，全球已有 18 个国家和地区将针灸纳入医疗保险体系，针灸的对外传播和国际交流方兴未艾。第二部分聚焦于针灸疗法的循证评价及优势特色。以世界卫生组织（WHO）颁布的针灸治疗适应证和全球首个针灸临床证据图谱为基础，整体为您展现针灸疗法治疗不同疾病的研究现状。通过梳理高质量系统评价证据，选取 10 种神经系统疾病，总结针灸治疗优势病种的有效性和安全性。临床实践指南是针对临床问题，基于证据的系统评价，并充分权衡不同干预措施利弊后，旨在为患者提供最佳医疗服务的推荐意见，本部分同时全面分析了针灸在临床实践指南中的推荐情况。针灸在临床实践指南中得到推荐，尤其是被国际期刊发表的临床实践指南推荐且为强推荐，更有助于推动针灸在临床实践和卫生决策领域的应用。第三部分将引领您探索针灸国际标准化的发展历程，并介绍针灸国际标准的制定现状，详细解读中方作为提案国主导研制的 8 项针灸 ISO 国际标准。针灸国际标准是世界范围内开展针灸临床实践和科学研究统一使用的技术“语言”，是在国际共识基础上经协商一致，可以共同使用和重复使用的规范性技术文件，共享相同的技术框架，能够有效推动针灸先进技术经验向全球传播、扩散，实现国际标准对全球针灸相关医疗资源的高效配置。

本书的编写人员以中国中医药循证医学中心和中国中医科学院中医临床基础医学研究所人员为主，并根据内容需求，邀请了来自针灸、中医医史文献、标准化等领域的专家参与，力求为读者提供一份全面而权威的针灸标准化和循证实践知识。本书在编写过程中得到了国家中医药管理局中医药标准化工作办公室的大力支持，在此深表感谢！本书的编写也得到了石学敏院士等专家的悉心指导，在此向各位中医前辈致敬！

在本书的编写过程中，我们深感责任重大，希望通过这部作品，能从标准和循证实践的角度为广大读者带来关于针灸的深入思考与启发。针灸不仅是中华传统医学的瑰宝，更是一门深邃而博大的医学科学。我们期待这本书能够激发您对针灸的兴趣，为您打开一个全新的医学视角。祝愿您在阅读的过程中获得充实的收获与启迪。

《针灸标准化与循证实践》编辑委员会

2023 年 12 月 1 日

FOREWORD

In modern medical practice, standardization and evidence-based medicine are two key pillars ensuring the quality of healthcare and driving medical progress. Standardization provides a common technical language, enabling medical practices from different regions and cultures to communicate and collaborate under the same standards. Evidence-based medicine, through systematic research and validation, ensures that medical decisions are based on the latest and most reliable scientific evidence. Acupuncture, as a traditional Chinese medical (TCM) treatment with a long history and widespread application, has made significant progress in standardization and evidence-based research. This combination of traditional wisdom and modern science has gradually integrated acupuncture into global medical practices, showcasing its unique value in different cultural and social contexts, and providing patients with safer and more reliable treatment options.

This book is divided into three parts. The first part takes you through a journey across millennia, delving into the evolution of acupuncture across different civilizations and eras, with a focus on important medical classics in the history of acupuncture civilization, including *the Yellow Emperor's Inner Classic (Huangdi Neijing), the Spiritual Axis (Lingshu Jing), the Classic of Difficult Issues (Nanjing), the Systematic Classic of Acupuncture and Moxibustion (Zhenjiu Jiayijing)* and others. We trace its origins, discuss its spread and development, and systematically outline how acupuncture has become a cross-border therapy and achieved remarkable achievements in the contemporary global context, from legislative, educational, and international exchange perspectives. To date, 18 countries and regions worldwide have incorporated acupuncture into their healthcare insurance systems, and its dissemination and international exchange continue to flourish. The second part focuses on the evidence-based evaluation and distinctive advantages of acupuncture therapy. Based on the indications for acupuncture treatment issued by the World Health Organization (WHO) and the world's first acupuncture clinical evidence map, this section presents the current state of research on acupuncture treatment for various diseases. By reviewing high-quality systematic review evidence and selecting ten neurological diseases, it summarizes the efficacy and safety of acupuncture treatment. Clinical practice guidelines are evidence-based systematic reviews aimed at addressing clinical questions and making balanced recommendations for patient care after weighing the pros and cons of different interventions. This section also comprehensively analyzes the recommendations of acupuncture in clinical practice guidelines, especially those strongly recommended by international journals, further promoting the application of acupuncture in clinical practice and health decision-making. The third part leads you to explore the development of acupuncture international standardization and introduces the current status of acupuncture international standards formulation, detailing the eight acupuncture ISO international standards led and developed by China as the proposer country. Acupuncture international standards are technical "languages" used uniformly in acupuncture clinical practice and scientific research worldwide, based on international consensus and can be used and reused consensually, sharing the same technical framework. They effectively promote the global dissemination and spread of advanced acupuncture techniques, achieving efficient allocation of global acupuncture-related medical resources.

The authors of this book are primarily from the China Center for Evidence Based Traditional Chinese Medicine and the Institute of Basic Research in Clinical Medicine, China Academy of Chinese Medical Sciences. According to content needs, experts from acupuncture, Chinese medical history and literature, and standardization fields were invited to contribute, aiming to provide readers with a comprehensive and authoritative knowledge of acupuncture standardization and evidence-based practice. The writing of this book was greatly supported by the Office of Traditional Chinese Medicine Standardization Administration of the National Administration of Traditional Chinese Medicine, for which we are deeply grateful. The writing also received meticulous guidance from experts such as Academician Shi Xuemin, to whom we pay our respects to all predecessors of Chinese medicine.

In the process of writing this book, we felt a great sense of responsibility and hope that this work can bring deep reflections and insights on acupuncture from the perspectives of standards and evidence-based practice to a wide range of readers. Acupuncture is not only a treasure of TCM but also a profound and extensive medical science. We hope this book will inspire your interest in acupuncture and open up a new medical perspective for you. We wish you a rewarding and enlightening reading experience.

Acupuncture Standardization and Evidence-based Practice editorial committee
December 1st , 2023

目录

三 针灸国际标准化

CONTENTS

一 针灸的历史发展及全球化进程

Chapter One
History of Acupuncture and Its Globalization Process

针灸由“针”和“灸”构成，是祖国医学的重要组成部分之一，其内容包括针灸理论、针灸技术、腧穴以及相关器具，在形成、应用和发展的过程中，具有鲜明的中华民族文化与地域特征，是基于中华民族文化和科学传统产生的宝贵遗产。

Acupuncture therapy, which is composed of “needling” (acupuncture) and “moxibustion”, is an integral part of traditional Chinese medicine, involving the theory of acupuncture and moxibustion, acupuncture and moxibustion techniques, acupoints, as well as related instruments. In the course of its formation, application, and development, acupuncture enjoys distinct cultural and regional characteristics of the Chinese nation, and is a precious heritage derived from the Chinese cultural and scientific tradition.

针法是指在中医理论的指导下把针具（通常指毫针）按照一定的角度刺入患者体内，运用捻转与提插等针刺手法来对人体特定部位进行刺激从而达到治疗疾病的目的。刺入点称为人体腧穴，简称穴位。

Acupuncture serves as a therapy which uses needles (usually filiform needles) under the guidance of traditional Chinese medicine theory to puncture the patient’s body at a certain angle. By applying rotating and lifting-thrusting techniques, it stimulates specific parts of the human body to achieve the purpose of treating the disease. The puncture point is called the body acupuncture point, the acupoint for short.

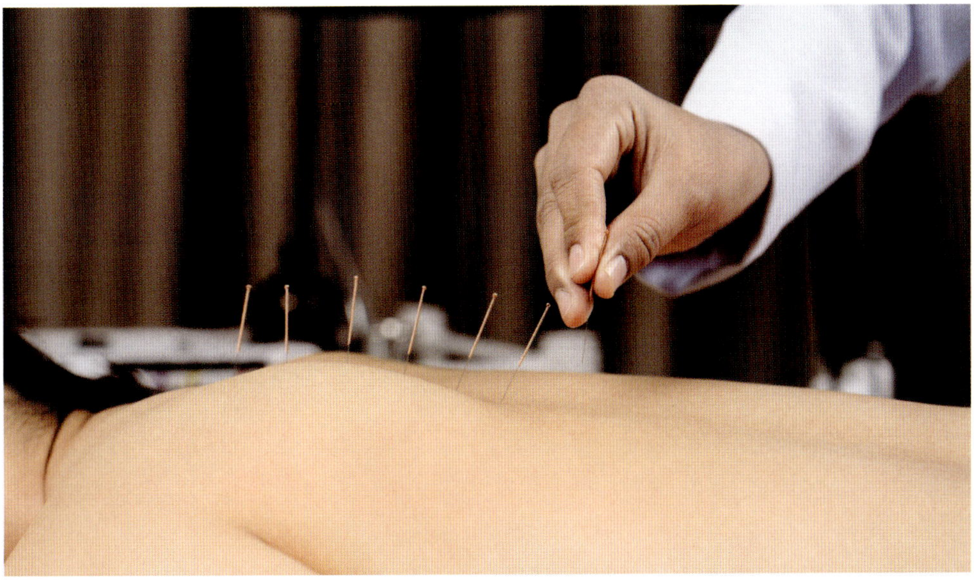

灸法是以预制的灸炷或灸条在体表一定的穴位上烧灼、熏熨，利用热的刺激来预防和治疗疾病。通常以艾草最为常用，故而称为艾灸，另有隔药灸、柳条灸、灯芯灸、桑枝灸等方法。

Moxibustion is a therapy which uses prefabricated moxa cones or moxa strips to burn, smoke and iron on certain points on the body surface to prevent and treat diseases with heat stimulation. Usually, wormwood is the most frequently utilized, so it is called moxibustion, and there are other alternative methods such as herbs-partitioned moxibustion, wicker moxibustion, burning rush moxibustion, and mulberry twig moxibustion.

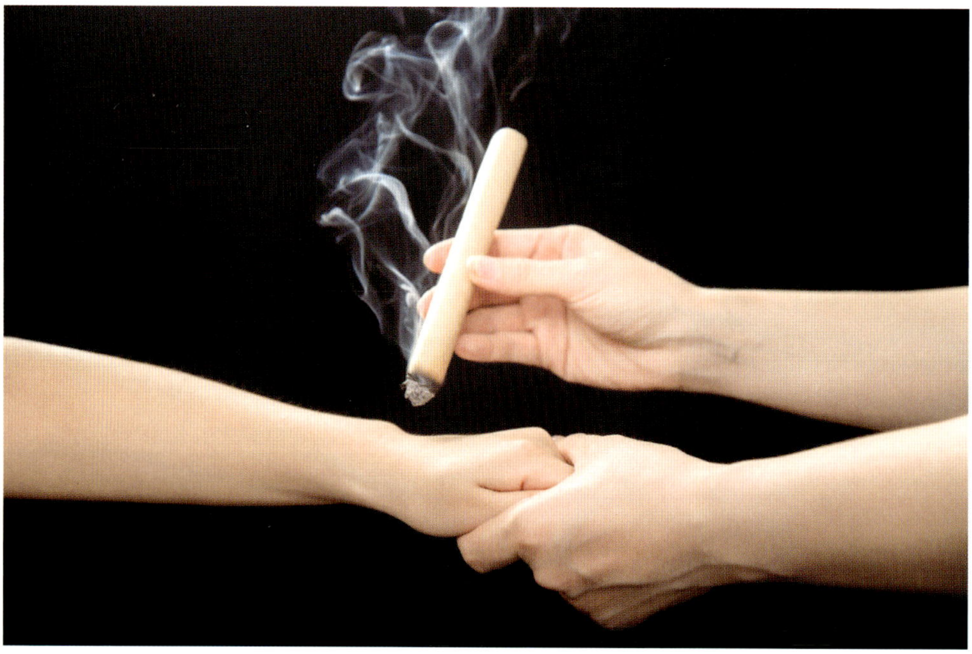

（一）针灸的发展简史
Part 1 A brief history of acupuncture

针灸，源自中国，有着数千年的历史，它结合了中医理论和独特的针灸技术，为人类的健康和治疗做出了巨大的贡献。

Originating from China, acupuncture dates back thousands of years. It has made great contributions to human health and medical treatment thanks to its combination of Chinese medical theories and unique acupuncture techniques.

1. 战国至秦汉时期
1. From the Warring States Period to the Qin and Han Dynasties

《黄帝内经》我国现存最早的医学经典著作，构筑起以经络学说为核心的针灸理论框架[1]，其中以《灵枢》所载针灸理论更为丰富和系统，故《灵枢》又称《针经》，为针灸学术的发展奠定了坚实的理论基础[2]。

The Yellow Emperor's Inner Classic (Huangdi Neijing), China's earliest surviving medical classics, set up a theoretical framework for acupuncture centered on the theory of science of channels and collaterals. *The Spiritual Pivot* (*Lingshu Jing)*, which features most extensive and systematic theories of acupuncture is also known as *The Classic of Acupuncture (Zhenjing)*, having laid a solid theoretical foundation for the academic development of acupuncture.

《难经》进一步补充了奇经八脉和原穴的论述，进一步丰富和充实了针灸学理论体系[3]。

[1] 傅维康 . 针灸发展史 [J]. 中国科技史料 ,1981(3):80-85.

[2] 辛智科 . 中国针灸医学发展史探 [J]. 陕西中医学院学报 ,1989(3):33-35.

[3] 何文菊 , 赵雪 , 陈泽林，等 . 古代针灸标准浅探 [C]// 中国针灸学会 . 2011 中国针灸学会年会论文集（摘要）. 2011:5.

The Classic of Difficult Issues (Nanjing) is a further supplement to the exposition of the eight extra meridians and the Yuan-primordial points, which further enriches and fleshes out the theoretical system of acupuncture.

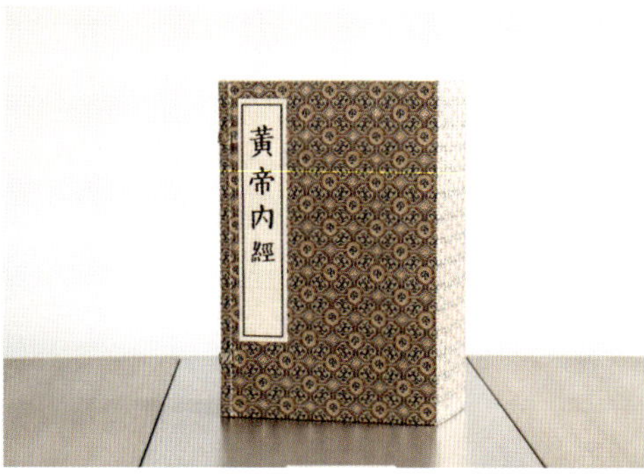

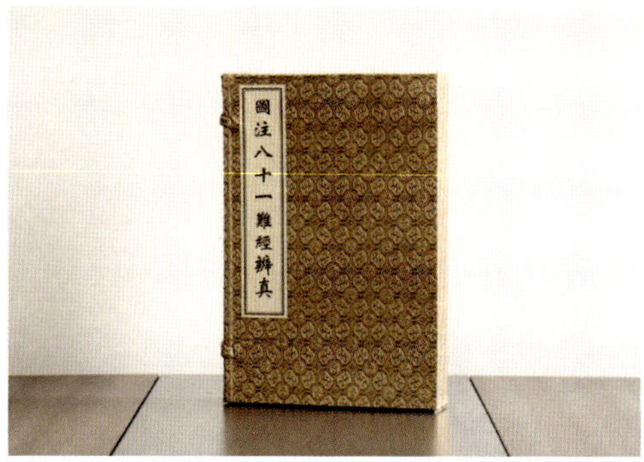

2. 魏晋隋唐时期

2. The Period from Wei, Jin, and Northern and Southern Dynasties to Sui and Tang Dynasties

皇甫谧的《针灸甲乙经》是现存的第一部针灸学专著，系统论述了有关脏腑、经络等理论，初步形成了经络、针灸理论[4]。也是继《黄帝内经》之后，对针灸医学的又一次总结，在针灸学发展史上起着承前启后的作用[5]。

Huangfu Mi's *The Systematic Classic of Acupuncture and Moxibustion (Zhenjiu Jiayijing)*, the first treatise on acupuncture in Chinese history, which systematically discusses the theories such as viscera and meridians, and initially forms the theory of meridians and acupuncture. As a successor to *The Yellow Emperor's Inner Classic (Huangdi Neijing)*, it summarizes acupuncture medicine, playing a role in the history of acupuncture.

[4] 辛智科 . 中国针灸医学发展史探 [J]. 陕西中医学院学报 ,1989(3):33-35.

[5] 王峰 , 赵中亭 .《针灸甲乙经》在针灸史上的重要地位 [J]. 山东中医药大学学报 ,2010,34(5):447-448.

孙思邈撰的《备急千金要方》，首载阿是穴法和指寸法[6]，广泛地收入了前代各家的针灸临床经验，并绘制了《明堂三人图》，成为历史上最早的彩色经络腧穴图（佚）。

Sun Simiao's *Important Formulas Worth a Thousand Gold Pieces for Emergency (Beiji Qianjin Yaofang)*, the first book to contain the Ashi Acupuncture Point method and the Finger-length measurement method, which extensively included the acupuncture clinical practices of various schools in the previous generations. Featuring *The Acupuncture and Moxibustion Chart (Mingtang Sanrentu)*, it was arguably the earliest colorful meridian acupoints chart in history (lost).

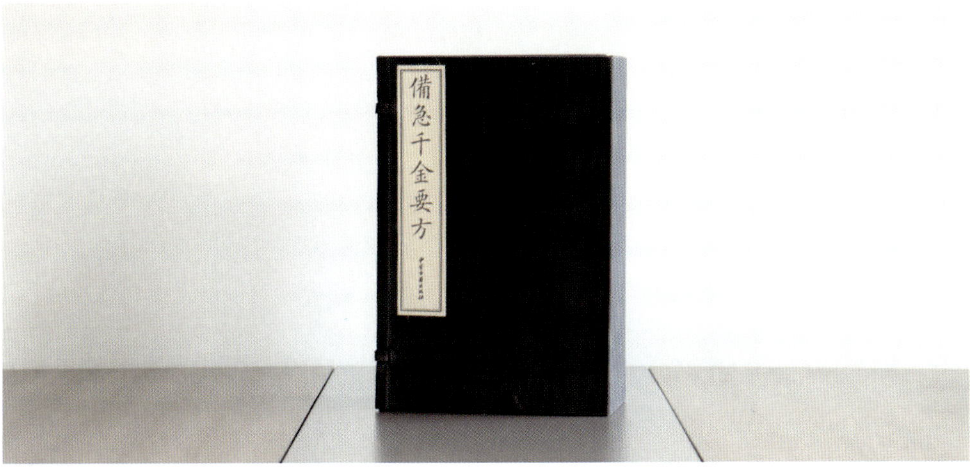

3. 宋金元时期

3. The Period of Song, Jin and Yuan Dynasties

北宋的王惟一撰写《铜人腧穴针灸图经》，并通过国家支持铸成针灸铜人模型两个，是世界上最早的立体针灸模型，开创经穴模型直观教学之先河[7,8]。

[6] 何文菊，赵雪，陈泽林，等．古代针灸标准浅探[C]// 中国针灸学会.2011 中国针灸学会年会论文集（摘要）. 2011:5.

[7] 中国非物质文化遗产：针灸[N]. 世界报,2008-07-16(017).

[8] 张五钢．漫谈北宋的针灸学[J]. 河南中医药学刊,1996(6):20-22.

Wang Weiyi of the Northern Song Dynasty authored the *Illustrated Classic of Acupoints on the Bronze Figure (Tongren Shuxue Zhenjiu Tujing)*. With the support of the Northern Song government, he cast two bronze figure models for acupuncture, the world's earliest three-dimensional model for acupuncture in existence, and pioneered the intuitive teaching with models for acupuncture and meridian points.

元代的滑寿，考订经络循行及其与腧穴的联系，撰写了《十四经发挥》，首次把任、督脉和十二经脉并称为“十四经”，进一步发展了经络腧穴理论[9]。

Thanks to a study of the circulation of meridians and their connection with acupoints, Hua Shou of the Yuan Dynasty authored the *Elucidation on Fourteen Channels (Shisijing Fahui)*, incorporating the Ren meridian and the Du meridian along with the twelve meridians as the Fourteen Meridians for the first time. Because of this work, the theory of meridians and acupoints was further developed.

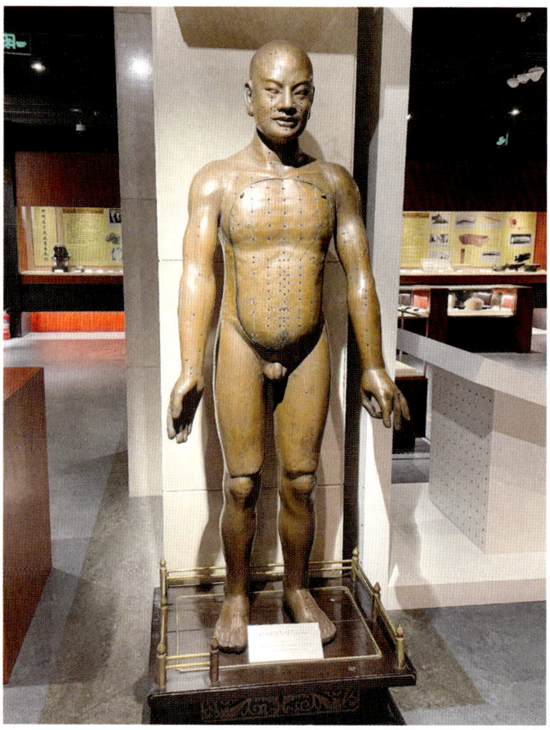

[9] 何文菊，赵雪，陈泽林，等．古代针灸标准浅探 [C]// 中国针灸学会 .2011 中国针灸学会年会论文集（摘要）. 2011:5.

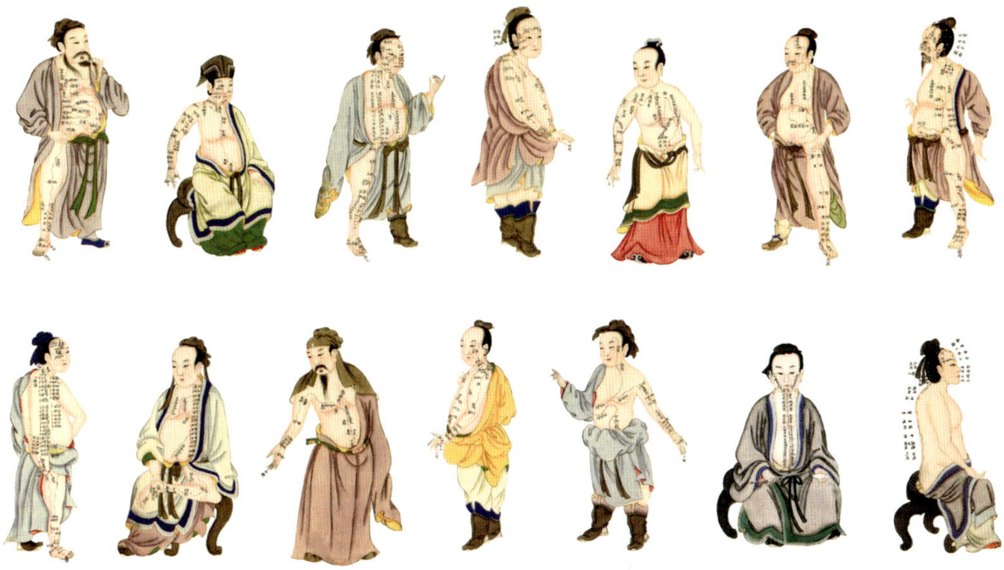

4. 明清时期

4. Ming and Qing Dynasties

明代针灸学术发展的主要表现：第一，对前代的针灸文献进行了广泛的搜集整理，出现了许多汇总历代针灸文献的著作，如：杨继洲的《针灸大成》[10]。第二，针灸手法的研究更加深入，在单式手法的基础上形成了二十多种复式手法。第三，对于历代不属于经穴的针灸部位进行了整理，在腧穴里列出“奇穴”这个类别[11]。

The Ming Dynasty saw a significant development in acupuncture. First, thanks to the efforts to collect and collate a wide range of acupuncture literature from previous generations, there appeared multiple works summarizing acupuncture literature from previous generations, such as Yang Jizhou's *The Great Compendium of Acupuncture and Moxibustion (Zhenjiu*

[10] 陈道瑾．试述明清时期针灸学的兴衰 [J]. 南京中医学院学报 ,1985(4):43-45.

[11] 梁繁荣 , 王华．针灸学 [M]. 北京：中国中医药出版社 ,2016.

Dacheng). Second, the deeper study of acupuncture techniques led to the formation of more than 20 types of compound techniques on the basis of single-type techniques. Third, the extra points were categorized as peculiar acupoints' following the classification of acupuncture points that did not belong to the extra points in the past.

从清初到鸦片战争这一历史时期，医者重药而轻针，针灸逐渐转入低谷。18 世纪吴谦等人奉敕撰《医宗金鉴・刺灸心法要诀》，以歌诀和插图为主，很切合实用[12]。

From the beginning of the Qing Dynasty to the Opium War period, doctors valued medication over acupuncture, accounting for the gradual decline of acupuncture. In the 18th century, Wu Qian and others, by order of the Imperial Decree, compiled the *Golden Mirror of the Medical Tradition · Essential Teaching on Acupuncture and Moxibustion (Yizong Jinjian-Cijiu Xinfa Yaojue)* . With mnemonic rhyme and illustrations, it is very practical.

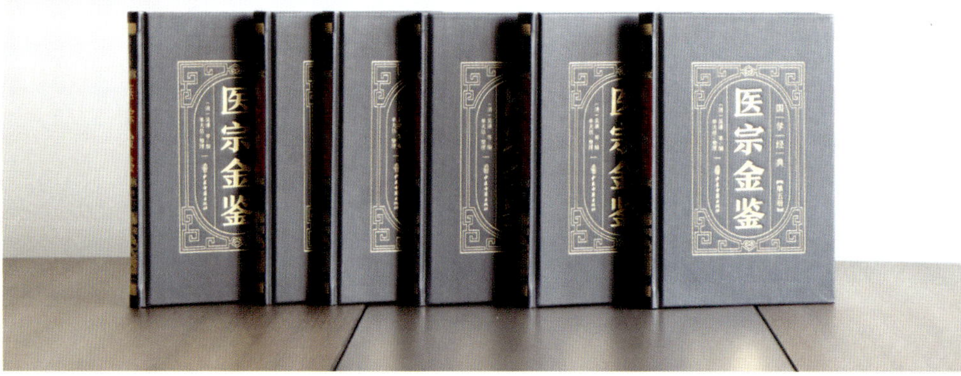

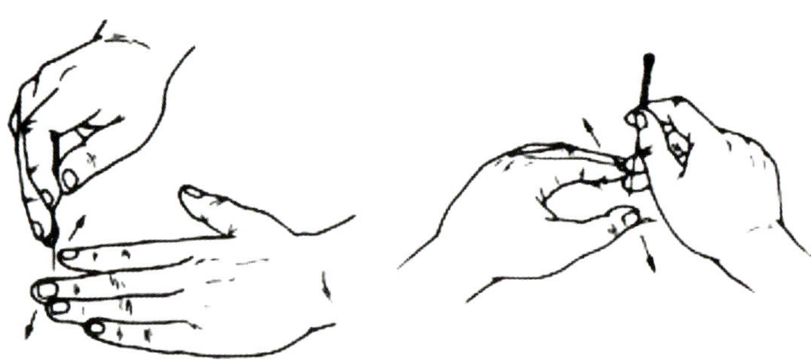

[12] 李嘉，徐恒泽 . 金元明清针灸歌赋述要 [J]. 南京中医药大学学报 ,1997(6):40-41.

（二）针灸的对外传播
Part 2 Global footprints of acupuncture

针灸的对外传播同样历史悠久，公元 6 世纪前后针灸传入周边的朝鲜半岛和日本，由此开始了迄今为止长达 1500 年之久的全球化之旅，时间之长和地域之广都是十分罕见的。纵观针灸对外传播的历史，大致可以划分为三个阶段[13]：

The international dissemination of acupuncture also goes back a long way. Since its introduction to the neighboring Korean Peninsula and Japan around the 6th century A.D., acupuncture has embarked on a journey of globalization that has lasted for 1500 years so far, which is rare in terms of both duration and geographical spread. Historically, the international spread of acupuncture and moxibustion can be roughly divided into three stages:

第一阶段：公元 6 世纪左右至 15 世纪末。针灸主要在中国周边地区，如朝鲜半岛、日本、越南、印度尼西亚等地区传播。

The first stage is from the 6th century A.D. to the end of the 15th century. Acupuncture was primarily spread in areas around China, such as the Korean Peninsula, Japan, Vietnam, and Indonesia.

第二阶段：公元 16 世纪初至 1970 年。早期主要传播到荷兰、法国、英国、德国、意大利等欧洲国家，并在 19 世纪初通过欧洲传播到美国、澳大利亚和俄罗斯等国。后期从 1963 年开始，中国政府派遣的援非医疗队将针灸传播到很多非洲国家。

The second stage was from the beginning of the 16th century to 1970. In the early period, it spread mainly to European countries such as the Netherlands, France, England, Germany, and Italy, and reached countries such as the United States, Australia, and Russia through Europe in the early 19th century. In the later period, starting from 1963, the Chinese government dispatched medical teams to aid Africa to spread acupuncture to many African countries.

[13] 白兴华 . 针灸对外传播的分期及各时期的特点 [J]. 中国针灸 ,2014,34(11):1141-1143.

第三阶段：1971 年至今。1971 年是个重要分水岭，《纽约时报》刊载了专栏记者赖斯顿撰写的其在中国北京做阑尾炎手术后接受针灸治疗的经历 [14]，此后形成一股世界性的“针灸热”，势不可挡，持续至今。

The third stage is from 1971 to present. A significant watershed year was 1971, when *The New York Times* published a story about the columnist Reston's experience with acupuncture after an appendicitis operation in Beijing, China, which led to the formation of a worldwide “acupuncture boom” that is unstoppable and lasts to this day.

世界卫生组织（World Health Organization，WHO）倡导针灸防治疾病，重视针灸的推广和交流。受 WHO 委托，中国于 1975 年在北京、南京、上海三地建立了国际针灸培训中心，每年开办国际针灸班，培养针灸人才。自 1963 年以来，中国政府坚持向非洲国家派出有针灸医师参与的援外医疗队，为这些国家培养了大批针灸医生，2023 年是中国援外医疗队派遣 60 周年。60 年来，中国累计向全球 76 个国家和地区派遣医疗队员 3 万人次，诊治患者 2.9 亿人次，赢得国际社会广泛赞誉 [15]。1979 年，WHO 提倡学习和应用针灸，并提出了适用针灸治疗的 43 种疾病的名称，予以推广，1996 年这个名单扩增至 64 种，2002 年进一步扩增到 107 种 [16,17]。在 WHO 的大力支持下，1987 年 11 月，世界针灸学会联合会在北京成立，负责国际针灸医师水平考核，为合格者颁发针灸医师水平证书，迄今已有 60 个国家和地区的 206 个会员团体。WHO 倡导针灸的标准化、规范化，制订了经穴名称、定位的国际标准化方案，以及头针的国际标准等。

The World Health Organization (WHO) advocates the use of acupuncture in the prevention and treatment of diseases, and attaches considerable importance to the promotion and communication of acupuncture. Entrusted by WHO, China established the International Acupuncture Training Center in Beijing, Nanjing and Shanghai in 1975, and offers international acupuncture training courses every year to cultivate acupuncture professionals. Since 1963, the Chinese government has continued its efforts to deploy medical aid teams

[14] RESTON J. Now about my operation In Peking [N]. The New York Times, 1971-01-26 (1,6).

[15] 中国政府网 . 习近平回信勉励援中非中国医疗队队员 [EB/OL]. (2023-12-12). https://www.gov.cn/xinwen/2023-02/10/content_5740961.htm.

[16] 茅骏霞 . 国外针灸临床研究现状文献分析 [J]. 江苏中医药 ,2019,51(7):54-58.

[17] WHO. Acupuncture: review and analysis of reports on controlled clinical trials [M]. Geneva: WHO, 2002 .

to African countries with the participation of acupuncturists, and has trained a large number of acupuncturists for these countries. This year (2023) marks the 60th anniversary of the Chinese Medical Teams (CMT) dispatched to foreign countries. Over the past 60 years, China has dispatched 30 000 CMT members to 76 countries and regions around the world, with a total of 290 million patients treated, garnering wide acclaim from the international community. In 1979, WHO advocated the study and application of acupuncture and proposed the names of 43 diseases where acupuncture could be applied and popularized, and this list was extended to 64 diseases in 1996, and further extended to 107 diseases in 2002. Under the auspices of WHO, the World Federation of Acupuncture-Moxibustion Societies (WFAS) was established in Beijing in November 1987, which is responsible for the international accreditation examination for acupuncture practitioners, and the issuance of certificates for qualified practitioners. So far there are 206 member groups from 60 countries and regions. WHO champions the standardization and normalization of acupuncture, and has developed an international standardization scheme for meridian point names and positioning, and an international standard for scalp acupuncture, among others.

2010 年 11 月 16 日，中国申报的“中医针灸”项目正式通过联合国教科文组织保护非物质文化遗产政府间委员会第五次会议审议，被列入“人类非物质文化遗产代表作名录”[18]。

On November 16, 2010, China's nomination of Acupuncture and Moxibustion of TCM passed the fifth meeting of the Intergovernmental Committee for the Safeguarding of the Intangible Cultural Heritage of the United Nations Educational, Scientific and Cultural Organization (UNESCO) and was inscribed on the Representative List of the Intangible Cultural Heritage of Humanity.

2017 年 1 月，国家主席习近平在日内瓦访问了世界卫生组织并会见了陈冯富珍总干事。习近平和陈冯富珍共同出席了中国向世界卫生组织赠送针灸铜人雕塑仪式，并为针灸铜人揭幕[19]。

In January 2017, President Xi Jinping visited WHO and met with Director-General Margaret Chen-Feng Fuzhen in Geneva. Xi and Margaret Chen-Feng Fuzhen attended a

---

[18] 中国政府网．“中医针灸”列入人类非物质文化遗产代表作名录 [EB/OL]. (2010-11-25)[2023-12-12]. https://www.gov.cn/gzdt/2010-11/25/content_1753422.htm.

[19] 人民政协网．习近平访问世界卫生组织并会见陈冯富珍总干事 [EB/OL]. (2017-01-19)[2023-12-12]. https://www.rmzxb.com.cn/c/2017-01-19/1294302.shtml.

ceremony to unveil a bronze acupuncture sculpture presented by China to the WHO.

据 WHO 统计，中医药已传播到 183 个国家和地区，其中有 103 个会员国认可使用针灸，29 个设立了传统医学的法律法规，18 个将针灸纳入医疗保险体系[20]。针灸的对外传播和国际交流方兴未艾。针灸不仅为人类防治疾病提供了一种有效的医疗方法和手段，而且为世界医学开拓了新的研究领域，并将为人类健康事业和世界医学发展做出更大贡献。

According to WHO statistics, traditional Chinese medicine has reached 183 countries and regions, of which 103 member states have recognized the use of acupuncture, 29 member states have established laws and regulations on traditional medicine, and 18 member states have put acupuncture into their health insurance systems. The spread of acupuncture and international exchanges is on the rise. Acupuncture is not only an effective medical method and means for human beings to prevent and treat diseases, but also breaks new ground for the world medicine, and will make greater contribution to the cause of human health and the development of the world medicine.

---

[20] WHO Traditional Medicine Strategy 2014—2023[EB/OL]. (2019-03-04)[2023-12-12]. https://apps.who.int/iris/bitstream/ha ndle/10665/92455/9789241506090_eng.pdf?sequence=1.

二 针灸疗法的循证评价及优势特色

Chapter Two Evidence-based Evaluation and Benefits of Acupuncture Therapy

（一）WHO 颁布的针灸治疗适应证
Part 1 Indications for acupuncture treatment as published by WHO

在 1980 年出版的《世界卫生·针灸专刊》中，WHO 提出并建议在全世界推广应用针灸治疗的 43 种适应证，包含头痛、偏头痛、三叉神经痛、面神经麻痹、中风后的轻度偏瘫、周围性神经疾患、小儿脊髓灰质炎后遗症、坐骨神经痛、神经性膀胱功能失调、遗尿、肋间神经痛在内的 17 种神经肌肉骨骼疾病（见表 1），占比约百分之四十[21]。随后在 2002 年，WHO 在《针灸临床研究报告的回顾与分析》的第三部分再次详细分析了针灸治疗病症的范围及疗效，列出了 77 种疾病推荐针灸治疗（见表 2），神经系统疾病仍然占比最高[22]。

In the *World Health-Special Issue on Acupuncture* published in 1980, WHO proposed and recommended 43 indications for which the use of acupuncture should be promoted worldwide. These include 17 types of neuromusculoskeletal disorders such as headache, migraine, trigeminal neuralgia, facial nerve palsy, mild hemiplegia after stroke, peripheral nerve disorders, pediatric post-polio sequelae, sciatica, neurogenic bladder dysfunction, enuresis, and intercostal neuralgia (see table 1), which account for about 40 percent of the total. In 2002, the WHO analyzed the range of conditions treated with acupuncture and its efficacy in detail again in the third part of the *Acupuncture: Review and Analysis of Reports on Controlled Clinical Trials*. There were 77 diseases for which acupuncture treatment was recommended (see table 2), with neurological disorders continuing to account for the largest number of cases.

[21] 胡金生 .WHO(世界卫生组织) 公布推广的针灸主治 43 种病症是哪些 ?[J]. 中医杂志 ,1989(8):57.

[22] World Health Organization. Acupuncture: review and analysis of reports on controlled clinical trials[M]. Geneva: World Health Organization, 2002.

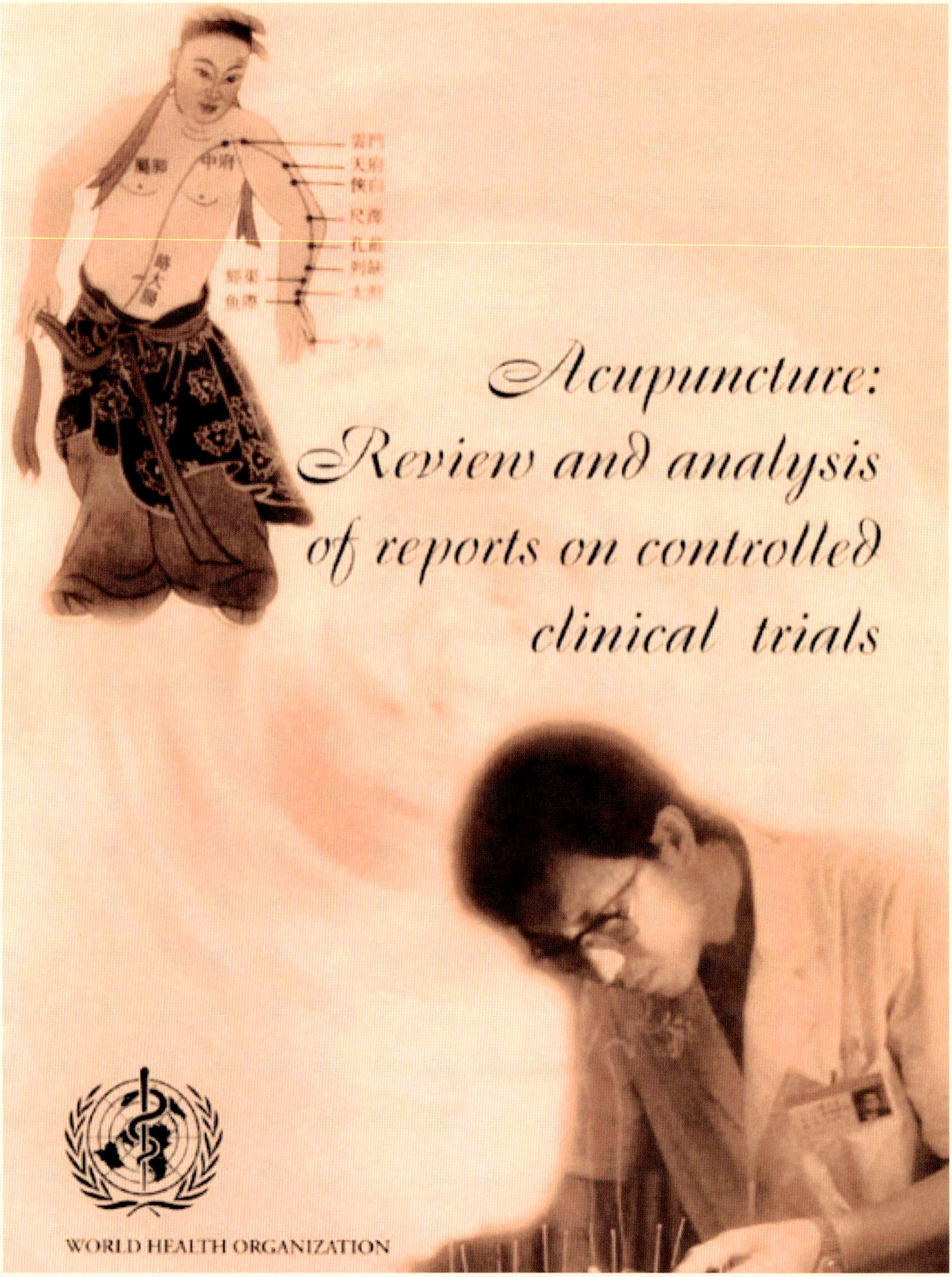
Acupuncture:
Review and analysis
of reports on controlled
clinical trials
WORLD HEALTH ORGANIZATION

表 1 《世界卫生 · 针灸专刊》(1980) 提及的 43 种针灸适应证
(Table 1 43 Kinds of Acupuncture Indication Mentioned in *World Health-Speial Issue* on Acupuncture in 1980)

针灸适应证	Indications for Acupuncture
上呼吸道疾病：1. 急性鼻窦炎，2. 急性鼻炎，3. 感冒，4. 急性扁桃腺炎	Upper respiratory tract diseases: 1. acute sinusitis, 2. acute rhinitis, 3. common cold, 4. acute tonsillitis
呼吸系统疾病：5. 急性气管炎，6. 支气管哮喘（对儿童和单纯性患者效果最佳）	Respiratory diseases: 5. acute bronchitis, 6. bronchial asthma (acupuncture is most effective for children and uncomplicated patients)
眼科疾病：7. 急性结膜炎，8. 中心性视网膜炎，9. 近视（儿童），10. 单纯性白内障	Ophthalmic diseases: 7. acute conjunctivitis, 8. central retinitis, 9. myopia (in children), 10. cataract (without complications)
口腔科疾病：11. 牙痛，12. 拔牙后疼痛，13. 牙龈炎，14. 急、慢性咽炎	Dental diseases: 11. toothache, 12. post extraction pain, 13. gingivitis, 14. acute and chronic pharyngitis
胃肠系统疾病：15. 食道、贲门痉挛，16. 呃逆，17. 胃下垂，18. 急、慢性胃炎，19. 胃酸过多，20. 慢性十二指肠溃疡（缓解疼痛），21. 单纯性急性十二指肠溃疡，22. 急、慢性结肠炎，23. 急性菌痢，24. 便秘，25. 腹泻，26. 肠麻痹	Diseases of the gastrointestinal system: 15. spasms of esophagus and cardia, 16. hiccough, 17. gastroptosis, 18. acute and chronic gastritis, 19. hyperacidity, 20. chronic duodenal ulcer (pain relief), 21. acute uncomplicated duodenal ulcer, 22. acute and chronic colitis, 23. acute bacillary dysentery, 24. constipation, 25. diarrhea, 26. paralytic ileus
神经、肌肉、骨骼疾病：27. 头痛，28. 偏头痛，29. 三叉神经痛，30. 面神经麻痹（早期如 3 ～ 6 个月之内者），31. 中风后的轻度瘫痪，32. 周围性神经疾患，33. 小儿脊髓灰质炎后遗症（早期如 6 个月之内），34. 梅尼埃病，35. 神经性膀胱功能失调，36. 遗尿，37. 肋间神经痛，38. 颈臂综合征，39. 肩周炎，40. 网球肘，41. 坐骨神经痛，42. 腰痛，43. 骨关节炎。	Neuromusculoskeletal disorders: 27. headache, 28. migraine, 29. trigeminal neuralgia, 30. facial palsy (within three to six months), 31. pareses following a stroke, 32. peripheral neuropathy, 33. sequelae of poliomyelitis (within six months), 34. Meniere's disease, 35. neurogenic bladder dysfunction, 36. enuresis, 37. intercostal neuralgia, 38. cervicobrachial syndrome, 39. periarthritis humeroscapularis, 40. tennis elbow, 41. sciatica, 42. low back pain, 43. osteoarthritis

表 2 《针灸临床研究报告的回顾与分析》(2002) 提及的 77 种针灸适应证
(Table 2 77 Kinds of Acupuncture Indications Mentioned in the *Acupuncture Review and Analysis of Reports on Controlled Clinical Trials* in 2002)

门诊常见病种	Common Outpatient Conditions
神经肌肉骨骼疾病：面瘫、中风、头痛、偏头痛、面肌痉挛、三叉神经痛、抽动——秽语综合征、小儿脑瘫、肩周炎、网球肘、坐骨神经痛、腰痛、风湿类风湿关节炎、膝关节疼痛、痛风性关节炎、肋间神经痛、纤维肌痛和筋膜炎、周围性神经疾患、强直性脊柱炎、神经性膀胱功能失调、梅尼埃病等	Neuromusculoskeletal disorders: facial paralysis, stroke, headache, migraine, facial spasm, trigeminal neuralgia, Tourette syndrome, pediatric cerebral palsy, periarthitis humeroscapularis, tennis elbow, sciatica, low back pain, rheumatoid arthritis, knee pain, gouty arthritis, intercostal neuralgia, fibromyalgia and fasciitis, peripheral neuropathy, ankylosing spondylitis, neurogenic bladder dysfunction, Meniere's disease, and so on
呼吸系统疾病：气管炎、支气管气喘、百日咳、急性鼻窦炎、急性鼻炎、感冒及急性扁桃腺炎等	Respiratory diseases: bronchitis, bronchial asthma, whooping cough, acute sinusitis, acute rhinitis, common cold and acute tonsillitis, and so on
消化系统疾病：食道痉挛、呃逆、胃动力功能障碍、消化不良、肠易激综合征、胃下垂、胃痛、急慢性浅表性胃炎、慢性萎缩性胃炎、急慢性十二指肠溃疡、单纯性急性十二指肠溃疡、消化不良、急慢性结肠炎、便秘、腹泻及肠麻痹等	Digestive diseases: esophageal spasm, hiccough, gastrokinetic disturbance, dyspepsia, irritable bowel syndrome, gastroptosis, epigastralgia, acute and chronic superficial gastritis, chronic atrophic gastritis, acute and chronic duodenal ulcers, acute uncomplicated duodenal ulcer, dyspepsia, acute and chronic colitis, constipation, diarrhea, paralytic ileus, and so on
泌尿系统疾病：女性尿道综合征、慢性前列腺炎、前列腺增生、遗尿、尿潴留（外伤）、尿路结石、遗尿等	Diseases of the urinary system: female urethral syndrome, chronic prostatitis, prostatic hyperplasia, enuresis, urinary retention (trauma), urolithiasis, enuresis, and so on

续表（continued table 2）

门诊常见病种	Common Outpatient Conditions
生殖系统疾病：月经不调、原发性痛经、更年期综合征、卵巢功能减退、多囊卵巢综合征、分娩痛、女性不孕、男子不育、产后缺乳、滞产、胎位不正等	Diseases of the reproductive system: irregular menstruation, primary dysmenorrhea, menopausal syndrome, hypoovarianism, polycystic ovary syndrome, labor pain, female infertility, male infertility, postpartum hypogalactia, stagnant labor, fetal malposition, and so on
其他：失眠、急性结膜炎、近视（儿童）、遗尿（小儿）牙痛、拔牙后疼痛、牙龈炎及急慢性咽炎、瘙痒症、肥胖、高脂血症、过敏性鼻炎、寻常痤疮、耳鸣耳聋、带状疱疹及后遗神经痛等	Others: insomnia, acute conjunctivitis, myopia (in children), enuresis (pediatrics), toothache, post extraction pain, gingivitis and acute and chronic pharyngitis, pruritus, obesity, hyperlipidemia, allergic rhinitis, acne vulgaris, tinnitus and deafness, herpes zoster, and postherpetic neuralgia, and so on
住院适应病种	**Conditions Requiring Hospitalization**
脑梗死急性期、恢复期、后遗症期，脑出血急性期、恢复期、后遗症期，截瘫、腰椎间盘突出症、肩周炎、颈椎病、面瘫、带状疱疹及后遗神经痛、强直性脊柱炎、单纯性肥胖等，三叉神经痛、周围性神经疾患、神经性膀胱功能失调、梅尼埃病等	Cerebral infarction in the acute stage, recovery stage, and sequelae stage; cerebral hemorrhage in the acute stage, recovery stage, and sequelae stage; paraplegia, lumbar intervertebral disc herniation, periarthritis of shoulder, cervical spondylosis, facial paralysis, herpes zoster and postherpetic neuralgia, ankylosing spondylitis, simple obesity, etc., trigeminal neuralgia, peripheral neuropathy, neurogenic bladder dysfunction, Meniere's disease, and so on

（二）全球首个针灸临床证据图谱
Part 2 The world’s first clinical evidence map for acupuncture

在 Web of Science 中检索，我们发现了 2471 篇针灸疗法的系统评价，在 2000 年至 2020 年期间，系统评价的数量逐年增加（见图 1）。已发表的关于随机试验（1578，63.9 %）和观察性研究（893，36.1 %）的系统评价主要集中在以下治疗领域：肌肉骨骼和结缔组织疾病（865，35.0 %），神经系统疾病（304，12.3 %），癌症（287，11.6 %），心血管疾病（235，9.5 %）[23]。

We identified 2471 systematic reviews of acupuncture therapies in the Web of Science between 2000 and 2020, with the number of systematic reviews increasing annually (see figure 1). Published systematic reviews of randomized trials (1578, 63.9%) and observational studies (893, 36.1%) mainly focused on the following therapeutic areas: musculoskeletal and connective tissue diseases (865, 35.0%), neurological conditions (304, 12.3%), cancer (287, 11.6%), and cardiovascular diseases (235, 9.5%).

纳入针灸系统评价（见图 2）的第一作者国别为中国（996，40.3 %），美国（358，14.5 %），英国（316，12.8 %），韩国（259，10.5 %），澳大利亚（178，7.2 %），加拿大（117，4.7 %），德国（106，4.3 %），其他（141，5.7 %）[23]。

The countries of the first author listed in acupuncture systematic reviews (see figure 2) were China (996, 40.3%), US (358, 14.5%), UK (316, 12.8%), South Korea (259, 10.5%), Australia (178, 7.2%), Canada (117, 4.7%), Germany (106, 4.3%), and elsewhere (141, 5.7%).

近 20 年来，随着人们对针灸疗法的认识和需求的不断增长，针灸的系统评价数量也在逐年稳步上涨。这些系统评价涵盖了针灸治疗各种疾病的效果、安全性和成本效益等方面的研究。通过系统评价，我们能够全面了解针灸在不同病种中的疗效，为临床医生和患者提供更加准确和可靠的决策依据（见图 3）。

[23] LU L, ZHANG Y, TANG X, et al. Evidence on acupuncture therapies is underused in clinical practice and health policy [J]. BMJ, 2022, 376: e067475.

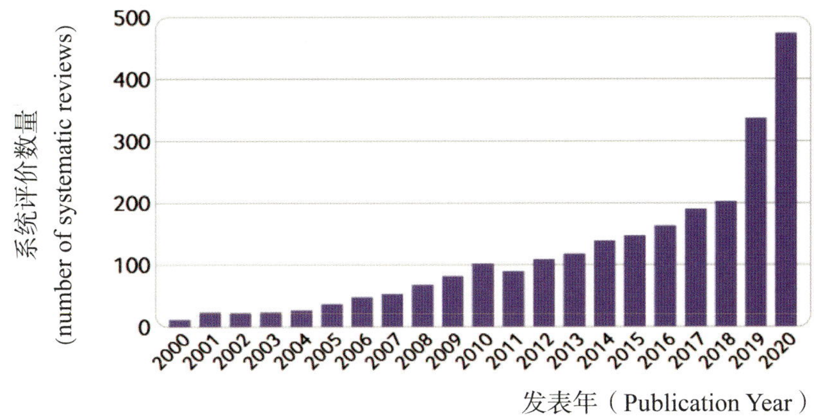

图 1　针灸系统评价发表年份图

（Figure 1　Publication Years of Systematic Review on Acupuncture）

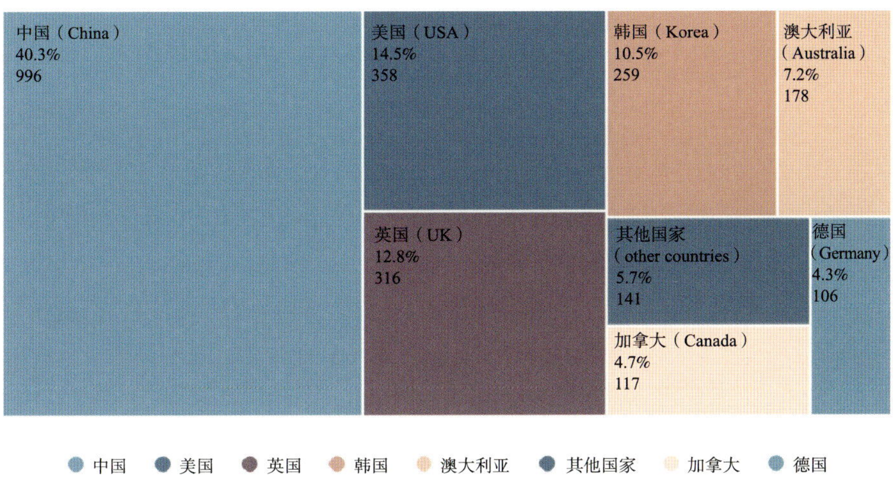

图 2　世界各国发表针灸系统评价数量占比图

（Figure 2　Proportion of Published Systematic Reviews on Acupuncture by Country）

As awareness of and demand for acupuncture therapy has been mounting over the past two decades, the number of systematic reviews of acupuncture has been steadily increasing year by year. These systematic reviews cover studies on the efficacy, safety and cost-effectiveness of acupuncture in the treatment of various diseases. The systematic reviews enables us to have a comprehensive understanding of the efficacy of acupuncture in different diseases and offers clinicians and patients a more accurate and reliable evidence for decision-making (see figure 3).

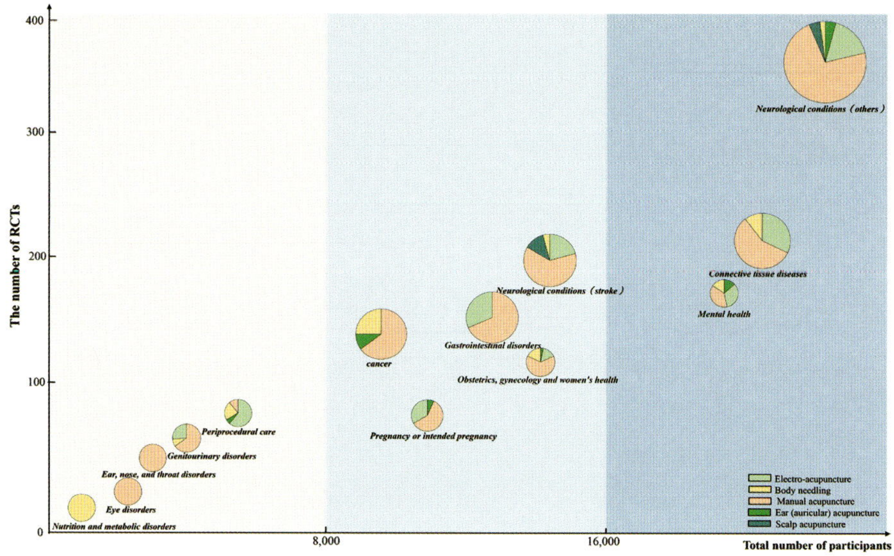

图 3　不同疾病的系统评价的 RCT 数量的气泡图

(Figure 3　Bubble Plot of the Number of RCTs in System Review of Different Diseases)

基于 1402 项随机对照试验研究和 138 995 名受试者的全球首个针灸证据图谱结果显示，针灸系统评价证据主要集中在 12 个疾病领域的 77 种病症(包括：围手术期护理、肿瘤学、神经病学、结缔组织病、耳鼻喉疾病、眼部疾病、胃肠道疾病、泌尿生殖系统疾病、精神健康、营养和代谢紊乱、产科、妇科和妇女健康，以及妊娠或计划妊娠)，其中神经系统疾病的针灸治疗证据最为丰富[24]。

According to the world's first evidence map of 1402 RCTs (ramdomized controlled trials) and 138 995 subjects, the results demonstrated that the evidence for the systematic review of acupuncture therapy mainly centered on 77 conditions in 12 disease domains, containing perioperative care, oncology, neurology, connective tissue disorders, ENT disorders, ocular disorders, gastrointestinal disorders, genitourinary disorders, mental health, nutritional and metabolic disorders, obstetrics, gynecology and women's health, and pregnancy or planned pregnancy, among which the evidence of acupuncture therapy for neurological diseases was the most abundant.

[24] LU L, ZHANG Y, GE S, et al. Evidence mapping and overview of systematic reviews of the effects of acupuncture therapies [J]. BMJ Open, 2022, 12(6):e056803.

（三）针灸疗法的优势疾病
Part 3 Main disease spectra of acupuncture

1. 抑郁症
1. Depression

1）针灸治疗抑郁症的机理
1) The mechanism of acupuncture in the treatment of depression

抑郁症是一种异质性疾病，具有多种病理生理机制，包括神经可塑性和炎症，进而产生各种症状模式。目前针对单一点的抑郁症药物治疗效果非常有限，抑郁症的标准药物治疗（主要是选择性血清素再摄取抑制剂，SSRIs）由于其不良反应和延迟起效，让患者不太满意。越来越多的证据表明，针灸加药物治疗比单独用药更有效、安全、耐受性好、起效早，这体现了针灸加药物治疗抑郁症的潜在益处。针灸治疗抑郁症的机制涉及多个生理和心理层面，已有研究表明其对神经递质、神经内分泌、免疫系统和心理状态的调节具有显著影响。针刺作为一种综合治疗抑郁症的手段，能够调节血清素和多巴胺的释放，有助于改善抑郁症状。此外，针灸还可通过抑制垂体—下丘脑—肾上腺轴的活动，减少应激激素的分泌，从而缓解抑郁症状。免疫学方面的研究表明，针灸对免疫系统产生调节作用，提高机体的抗炎水平，有助于缓解抑郁引起的身体不适感。此外，针灸还通过影响脑电图和脑功能成像结果，调整患者的心理状态，减轻焦虑和改善睡眠[25]。因此，针灸可能是对由多种机制引起的重度抑郁症的比较有潜力的治疗方法。

Depression is a heterogeneous disorder with various pathophysiological mechanisms, including neuroplasticity and inflammation, giving rise to diverse symptom patterns. Currently, the efficacy of antidepressant medications targeting specific points for depression is quite limited. Standard drug treatment for depression, mainly selective serotonin reuptake

[25] YANG NN, LIN LL, LI YJ, et al. Potential mechanisms and clinical effectiveness of acupuncture in depression [J]. Curr Neuropharmacol, 2022, 20(4): 738-750.

inhibitors (SSRIs), is often dissatisfactory due to adverse effects and delayed onset of action. Increasing evidence suggests that acupuncture combined with medication is more effective, safer, better tolerated, and faster acting than medication alone, highlighting the potential benefits of acupuncture in treating depression. The mechanism of acupuncture in treating depression involves multiple physiological and psychological aspects, with studies indicating significant modulation of neurotransmitters, neuroendocrine function, the immune system, and psychological states. Acupuncture, as a comprehensive treatment approach for depression, regulates the release of serotonin and dopamine, contributing to the improvement of depressive symptoms. Furthermore, acupuncture inhibits the activity of the hypothalamus-pituitary-adrenal axis, reducing the secretion of stress hormones and alleviating depressive symptoms. Immunological research suggests that acupuncture exerts a regulatory effect on the immune system, enhancing the body’s anti-inflammatory levels and helping to alleviate the physical discomfort associated with depression. Additionally, acupuncture adjusts patients’ psychological states, reduces anxiety, and improves sleep through its impact on electroencephalography and functional brain imaging. Therefore, acupuncture may be a promising therapeutic approach for severe depression with multiple underlying mechanisms.

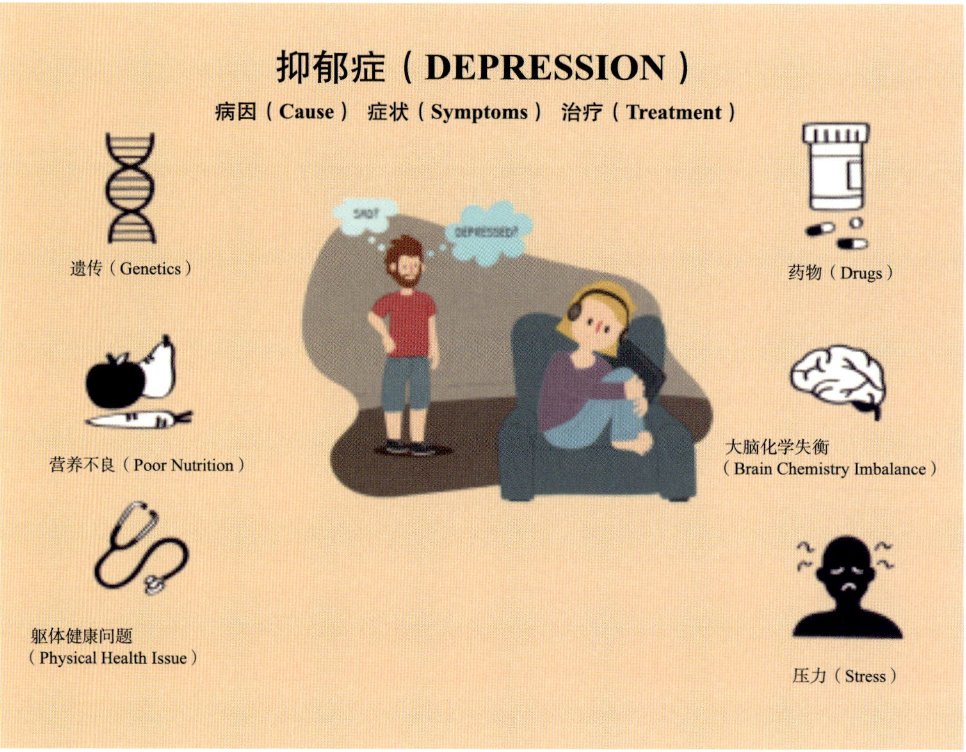

2）针灸治疗抑郁症临床疗效循证评价

2) Systematic evaluation of clinical effect of acupuncture on depression

2018 年，一项纳入了 64 项随机对照试验，涉及 7104 例患者的 Cochrane 系统评价 [26] 显示，与对照针灸（包括假针灸、最小针灸、模拟电针等）或无治疗相比，针灸治疗更能降低抑郁症严重程度。但很少有研究包括随访期或评估生活质量等重要结果。因此，迫切需要高质量的随机对照试验来检验针灸与对照针灸、药物治疗或心理治疗相比的有效性和可接受性（见表 3）。

In 2018, a Cochrane systematic review included 64 RCTs involving 7104 patients with depression showed: the reduction in severity of depression was more when acupuncture was compared with control acupuncture or no treatment control. But few studies involved follow-up periods or assessing important outcomes such as quality of life etc. Therefore, high-quality randomized controlled trials are urgently needed to examine the clinical efficacy and acceptability of acupuncture, as well as its effectiveness, compared with acupuncture controls, medication, or psychological therapies (see table 3).

表 3　针灸治疗抑郁临床疗效循证评价证据总结表

改善指标	对照类型	纳入研究数量	纳入患者数量		MD/SMD (or RR)（95%CI）	GRADE证据分级
			试验组	对照组		
抑郁严重程度	针灸 vs 空白对照 / 等待名单 / 常规治疗 [1]	5	237	251	SMD: −0.66(−1.06 to −0.25)	低等
	针灸 vs 药物 [1]	31	1598	1529	SMD: −0.23(−0.40 to −0.05)	极低等
	针灸 vs 对照针灸 [2]	14	368	473	MD: −1.69(−3.33 to −0.05)	低等
	针灸 + 药物 vs 药物 [1]	11	480	333	SMD: −1.15(−1.63 to −0.66)	极低等
	针灸 vs 心理治疗 [1]	2	173	324	SMD: 0.5(1.33 to 0.33)	低等

[26] SMITH CA, ARMOUR M, LEE MS, et al. Acupuncture for depression [J]. Cochrane Database Syst Rev, 2018, 3(3):CD004046.

续表

改善指标	对照类型	纳入研究数量	纳入患者数量		MD/SMD (or RR)（95%CI）	GRADE证据分级
			试验组	对照组		
不良反应	针灸 vs 空白对照 / 等待名单 / 常规治疗 *	1	151	151	RR: 0.89(0.35 to 2.24)	低等
	针灸 vs 药物[3]	3	237	244	MD: −4.32(−7.41 to −1.23)	极低等
	针灸 vs 对照针灸 *	5	158	142	RR: 1.63(0.93 to 2.86)	中等等
	针灸 + 药物 vs 药物 *[4]	3	100	100	SMD: −1.32(−2.86 to 0.23)	极低等
	针灸 vs 心理治疗 *	1	151	302	RR: 0.62(0.29 to 1.33)	低等

注: CI，置信区间；SMD，标准平均差；MD，平均差；RR，风险比。1，抑郁严重程度评估——采用多种医护人员或者自评工具进行的评价（分数越低，代表严重程度越低）。2，干预结束时抑郁症严重程度，以汉密尔顿抑郁量表（HAMD）评分 0 ～ 54 分（得分越低表示抑郁症越轻）。3，用 Asberg 抗抑郁药副作用量表进行测量。4，用 Asberg 抗抑郁药副作用量表和毒性暴露监测系统进行测量。* 为针灸和常规药物之间没有统计学差异。

Table 3　Summary of Evidence for the Effectiveness of Acupuncture in the Treatment of Depression

Outcomes	Comparison	No. of Studies	No. of Patients		MD/SMD (or RR) (95%CI)	Certainty of the Evidence (GRADE)
			T	C		
Severity of Depression	Acupuncture vs No Treatment/ Wait List/ Treatment as Usual[1]	5	237	251	SMD: −0.66 (−1.06 to −0.25)	Low
	Acupuncture vs Medication[1]	31	1598	1529	SMD: −0.23 (−0.40 to −0.05)	Very Low
	Acupuncture vs Co-ntrol Acupuncture[2]	14	368	473	MD: −1.69 (−3.33 to −0.05)	Low
	Acupuncture Plus Medication vs Medication[1]	11	480	333	SMD: −1.15 (−1.63 to −0.66)	Very Low

continued table 3

Outcomes	Comparison	No. of Studies	No. of Patients		MD/SMD (or RR) (95%CI)	Certainty of the Evidence (GRADE)
			T	C		
Severity of Depression	Acupuncture vs Psychological Therapy [1]	2	173	324	SMD: 0.5 (1.33 to 0.33)	Low
Adverse Events	Acupuncture vs No Treatment/ Wait List/ Usual Treatment*	1	151	151	RR: 0.89 (0.35 to 2.24)	Low
	Acupuncture vs Medication [3]	3	237	244	MD: −4.32 (−7.41 to −1.23)	Very Low
	Acupuncture vs Control Acupuncture*	5	158	142	RR: 1.63 (0.93 to 2.86)	Moderate
	Acupuncture Plus Medication vs Medication* [4]	3	100	100	SMD: −1.32 (−2.86 to 0.23)	Very Low
	Acupuncture vs Psychological Therapy* [5]	1	151	302	RR: 0.62 (0.29 to 1.33)	Low

Note: CI, confidence interval; SMD, standardized mean difference; MD, mean difference; RR, risk ratio; T, treatment group; C, control group. 1, Severity of depression assessed with various clinician-rated and self-rated outcome measures (lower score indicates less severe depression). 2, Severity of depression at the end of the intervention as measured by the Hamilton Depression Rating Scale (HAMD) scored from 0 to 54 (lower score indicates less severe depression). Comparisons are made between invasive and non-invasive controls. Invasive controls included non-channel points, needling acupuncture points unrelated to depression, minimal insertion just into the skin layer, different acupuncture points, and minimal insertion on specific non-depression points. Non-invasive controls included placebo needles, mock electro-acupuncture, and mock laser acupuncture. 3, measured with Asberg Antidepressant Side Effect Scale. 4, measured with Asberg Antidepressant Side Effect Scale and Toxic Exposure Surveillance System. 5, measured during study treatment. * There was no statistical difference between acupuncture and the conventional medicine.

3）针灸治疗抑郁症循证指南推荐
3) Clinical guideline recommendations for acupuncture in the treatment of depression

当前很多临床试验显示针灸治疗抑郁症有效，虽为低质量证据，但由于其治疗的潜力及安全性，因此，早在 2009 年针灸就被加拿大写入抑郁症管理指南中。并且有 2 项指南（分别由世界卫生组织传统医学办公室和加拿大精神病协会负责制定）明确推荐了针灸用于抑郁症的治疗 [27]。针灸治疗抑郁症临床指南推荐意见总结见图 4。

Many clinical trials showed that acupuncture is effective in the treatment of depression, although the evidence is of low quality. However, due to its potential and safty, acupuncture has been included in the Canadian Clinical guidelines for the management of major depressive disorder in adults as early as 2009. Moreover two guidelines have explicitly recommended acupuncture for the treatment of depression. Summary of clinical guideline recommendations for acupuncture in the treatment of depression is shown in figure 4.

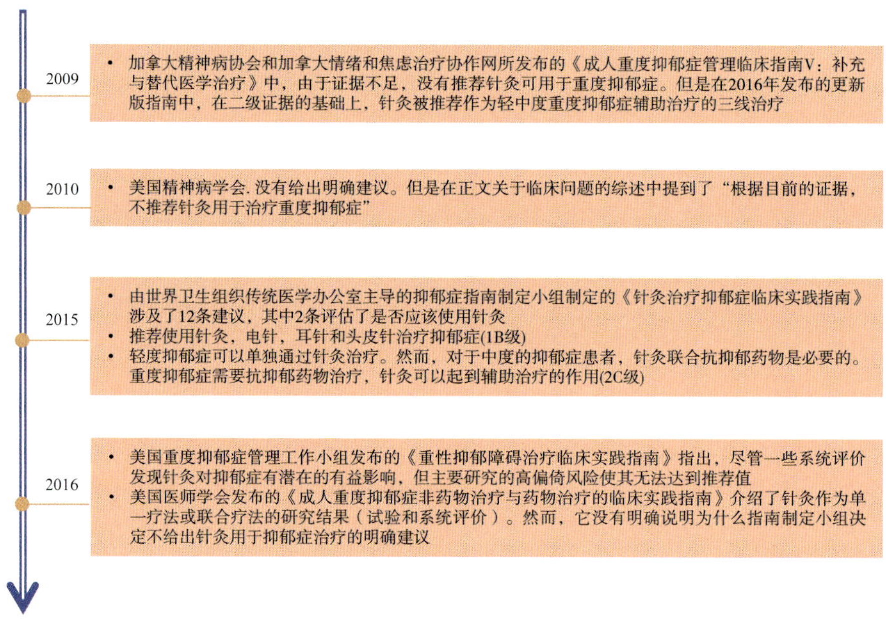

图 4　针灸治疗抑郁症临床指南推荐意见总结

[27] FERNANDE-CHINGUE JE, GOICCHEA-LUGO S, VILLARREA-ZEGARRA D, et al. Acupuncture for major depressive disorder: A review of the recommendations stated at clinical practice guidelines [J]. Complement Ther Med, 2020, 49: 102321.

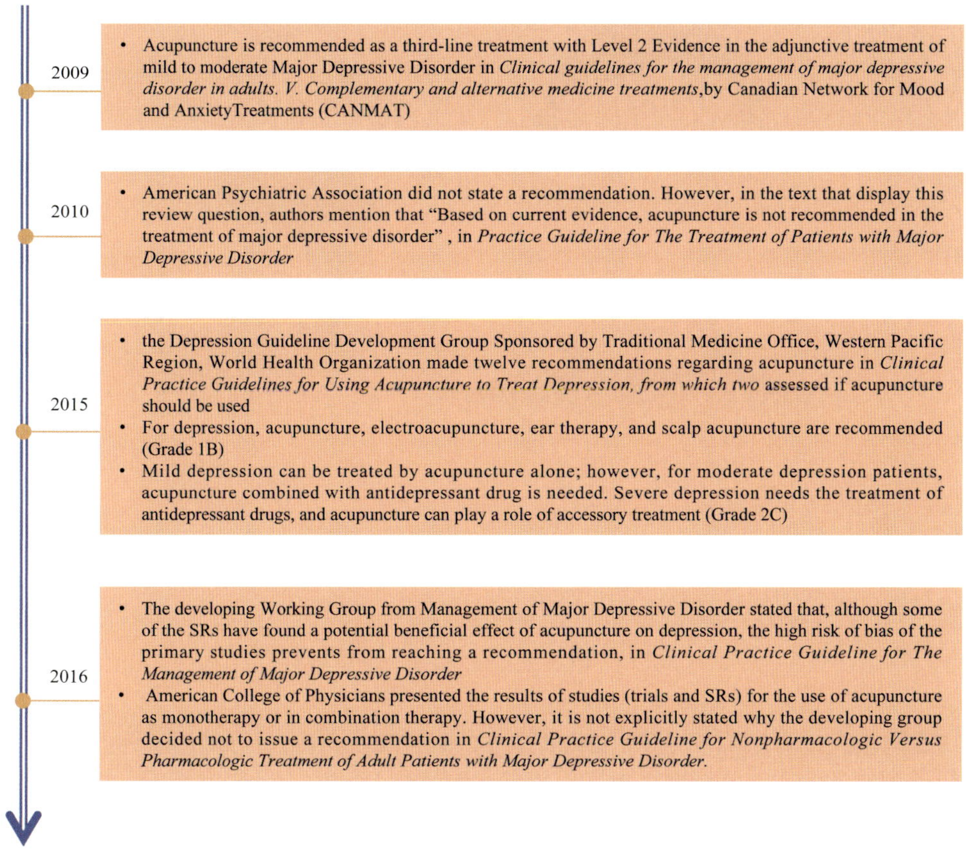

Figure 4 Summary of Clinical Guideline Recommendations for Acupuncture in the Treatment of Depression

2. 面瘫

2. Facial paralysis

1）针灸治疗面瘫的机理

1) The mechanism of acupuncture in the treatment of facial paralysis

面瘫是由于中枢性或周围性面神经疾病或损伤所致的面部肌肉神经性瘫痪，以口角向一侧歪斜、眼睑闭合不全为主症的病证。本病可发生于任何年龄，无明显的季节性，发病急，多见一侧面部发病。其发生常与劳作过度、正气不足、风寒或风

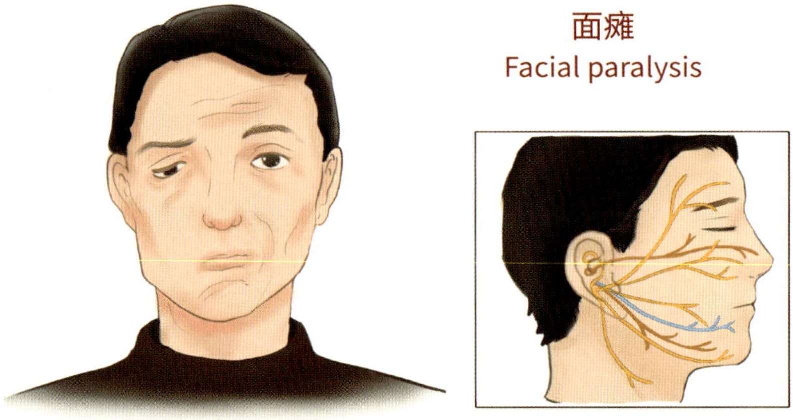

面瘫
Facial paralysis

热乘虚而入等因素有关。本病病位在面部，与少阳、阳明经筋相关[28]。针灸是国际上广泛使用的补充和替代治疗方法，已被证明对周围神经病变有显著疗效，世界卫生组织强烈建议使用针灸治疗面瘫[29]。现代科学为针灸的效果提供了生物学证据，揭示了针灸治疗（包括电针灸）最终可以通过激活周围神经通路来调节生理功能[30]。电针疗法通过针灸结合电刺激，有节奏地放松局部肌肉，更好地调节组织细胞功能，加强血液淋巴循环和离子运动，加速废物代谢，增加组织营养，消除炎症性水肿，从而促进受损神经和肌肉的修复和再生[31]。此外，针灸还可以促进轴突生长，调节血管收缩或血流动力学，并最终恢复受损面神经的功能[32]。

Facial paralysis is a symptom of crooked corners of the mouth to one side and incomplete closure of the eyes and face, also known as "crooked mouth and eyes". This disease can occur at any age, characterized with no obvious seasonality, acute symptoms, and mostly happens on one side of the face. It is often associated with overwork, lack of vital energy, wind-induced cold or heat and other factors. The disease manifests on the facial area and is related to the Shaoyang and Yangming meridians and tendons. Acupuncture is a widely used complementary and

[28] 梁繁荣，王华．针灸学 [M]. 北京：中国中医药出版社 ,2016:212.

[29] ZHANG YQ, LU L, XU N, et al. Increasing the usefulness of acupuncture guideline recommendations [J]. BMJ, 2022, 376: e070533.

[30] LIU S, WANG Z, SU Y, et al. A neuroanatomical basis for electroacupuncture to drive the vagal-adrenal axis [J]. Nature, 2021, 598(7882): 641-645.

[31] ZHAO MY, WANG PM. Progress of acupuncture and moxibustion in treatment of obstinate facial paralysis [J]. Clin J Tradit Chin Med, 2018, 30(9): 1757-1760.

[32] ZHOU X, XIONG J, CHI Z, et al. Effectiveness and safety of acupuncture and moxibustion for peripheral facial paralysis: A protocol for an overview of systematic reviews and meta-analysis [J]. Medicine (Baltimore), 2020, 99(38): e22371.

alternative treatment internationally and has been shown to have significant efficacy in peripheral neuropathy. The World Health Organization strongly recommends the use of acupuncture for the treatment of facial paralysis. Modern science has provided biological evidence for the effectiveness of acupuncture, revealing that acupuncture treatments [including electro-acupuncture (EA)] can ultimately regulate physiological functions by activating peripheral nerve pathways. EA can be combined with current stimulation through acupuncture and moxibustion to rhythmically relax local muscles, better regulate tissue cell function, strengthen blood lymphatic circulation and ion movement, accelerate waste metabolism, increase tissue nutrition, eliminate inflammatory edema, and thus promote the repair and regeneration of damaged nerves and muscles. In addition, it can promote axonal growth, regulate vasoconstriction or hemodynamics, and ultimately restore the function of the damaged facial nerve.

2）针灸治疗面瘫临床疗效循证评价
2) Systematic evaluation of clinical effect of acupuncture on facial paralysis

2023 年，一项纳入 18 个随机对照试验，共涉及 1118 名面瘫参与者的系统评价[33]显示：电针治疗比非电针治疗更能有效地提高总有效率，且亚组分析显示，电针治疗的总有效率也高于手针治疗。并且电针治疗比非电针治疗在提升治愈率、改善 Portmann 评分中均有显著优势。因此，建议根据不同的疾病时期选择不同的针灸治疗模式，在面瘫中后期提前使用电针，可能对患者有所帮助（见表 4）。

In 2023, a systematic review that included 18 RCTs involving a total of 1118 participants suggested that EA was more effective than non-EA treatment in increasing the overall effective rate, and subgroup analyses showed that EA was also more effective than manual acupuncture (MA). And EA had a significant advantage over non-EA in enhancing the cure rate and improving the Portmann score. It also suggested that different acupuncture treatment modes should be selected according to different disease periods, and EA should be used in advance in the middle and late stage of facial paralysis, which might be helpful for patients (see table 4).

[33] ZHOU Y, DONG X, XING Y, et al. Effects of electroacupuncture therapy on intractable facial paralysis: A systematic review and meta-analysis [J]. PLoS One, 2023, 18(7): e0288606.

表 4 针灸治疗面瘫临床疗效循证评价证据总结表

改善指标	对照类型	纳入研究数量	纳入患者数量		SMD（或 RR）(95%CI)	GRADE 证据分级
			试验组	对照组		
总有效率	电针 vs 常规药物	18	574	545	RR：1.23 (1.17 to 1.31)	中等
	电针 vs 手针	12	360	347	RR：1.26 (1.17 to 1.35)	中等
治愈率	电针 vs 常规药物	18	574	545	RR：2.04 (1.70 to 2.44)	中等
Portmann 评分	电针 vs 常规药物	3	72	72	SMD：1.32 (0.24 to 2.40)	低等

注：SMD，标准平均差；RR，风险比；CI，置信区间。

Table 4 Summary of Evidence for the Effectiveness of Acupuncture in the Treatment of Facial Paralysis

Outcomes	Comparison	No. of Studies	No. of Patients		SMD (or RR) (95%CI)	Certainty of the Evidence (GRADE)
			T	C		
Total Effective Rate	Electroacupuncture vs Conventional Medicine	18	574	545	RR: 1.23 (1.17 to 1.31)	Moderate
	Electroacupuncture vs Manual Acupuncture	12	360	347	RR: 1.26 (1.17 to 1.35)	Moderate
Cure Rate	Electroacupuncture vs Conventional Medicine	18	574	545	RR: 2.04 (1.70 to 2.44)	Moderate
Portmann Scores	Electroacupuncture vs Conventional Medicine	3	72	72	SMD: 1.32 (0.24 to 2.40)	Low

Note: SMD, standardized mean difference; RR, risk ratio; CI, confidence interval; T, treatment group; C, control group.

3）针灸治疗面瘫循证指南推荐

3) Clinical guideline recommendations for acupuncture in the treatment of facial paralysis

截至 2023 年 10 月，在 PubMed 中共检索到 3 篇关于面瘫英文指南中提及针灸治疗。其中，早在 2009 年，成都中医药大学团队发表了 *Evidence based acupuncture practice recommendations for peripheral facial paralysis* [34]，对针灸治疗的穴位选择、针刺手法进行了说明，将针灸治疗面瘫的有效性向世界展现，对贝尔麻痹治疗提供新的科学指导，推荐全球医生在治疗贝尔麻痹时，考虑针刺疗法。随后，在 2013 年，*Clinical practice guideline: Bell's palsy* [35] 在全球范围内发布，对针灸治疗贝尔麻痹进行标准化、规范化，推动针灸治疗的普及和认可，为国际交流提供了机会。该指南对贝尔麻痹的急性期、亚急性期、恢复期、后遗症期各个时期的选穴和刺法进行了规范，至今仍然适用。2019 年，在韩国出版了 *Clinical practice guideline of Korean Medicine: Facial palsy*[36]，针灸治疗贝尔麻痹逐渐被世界认可。针灸治疗面瘫的临床指南推荐意见总结见图 5。

As of October 2023, a total of 3 guidelines on facial palsy mentioned acupuncture treatment. As early as 2009, a team from Chengdu University of Traditional Chinese Medicine published *Evidence Based Acupuncture Practice Recommendations for Peripheral Facial Paralysis*, which explained the selection of acupuncture points and needling techniques for acupuncture treatment, presented the effectiveness of acupuncture treatment for facial palsy to the world, provided new scientific guidance for Bell's palsy treatment, and recommended that physicians worldwide consider acupuncture therapy when treating Bell's palsy. Subsequently, in 2013, *Clinical Practice Guideline of Acupuncture for Bell's Palsy* was released globally to standardize and regulate the treatment of Bell's Palsy with acupuncture, to promote the popularity and recognition of acupuncture treatment, and to provide a platform for international exchange. The guideline standardized the selection of points and stabbing methods for each period of Bell's palsy, including the acute, subacute, recovery, and sequelae phases, and is still applicable today. In 2019, in Korea, *the Clinical practice guideline of Korean Medicine:*

[34] ZHENG H, LI Y, CHEN M. Evidence based acupuncture practice recommendations for peripheral facial paralysis [J]. Am J Chin Med, 2009, 37(1): 35-43.

[35] BAUGH RF, BASURA GJ, ISHII LE, et al. Clinical practice guideline: Bell's palsy [J]. Otolaryngol Head Neck Surg, 2013, 149(3 Suppl): S1-S27.

[36] Guideline Center for Korean Medicine. Clinical practice guideline of Korean Medicine: Facial palsy 2018.

Facial palsy was published, and acupuncture for Bell's palsy was gradually being recognized worldwide. Summary of clinical guideline recommendations for acupuncture in the treatment of facial paralysis is shown in figure 5.

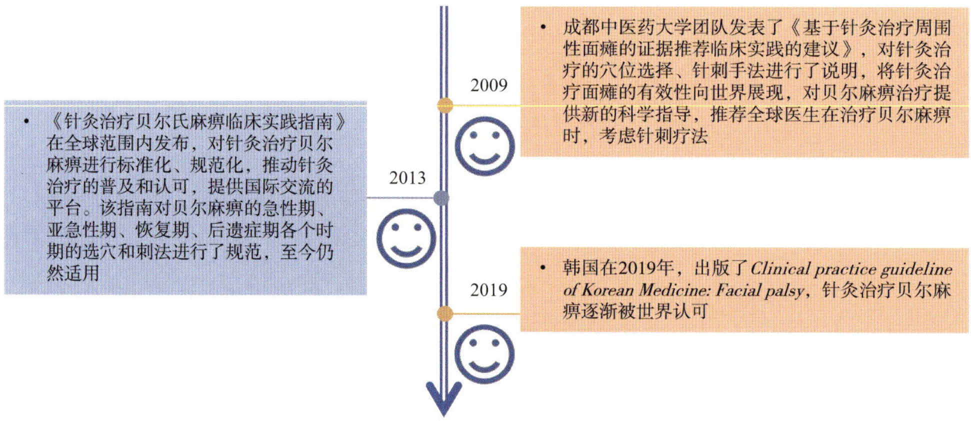

图 5　针灸治疗面瘫的临床指南推荐意见总结

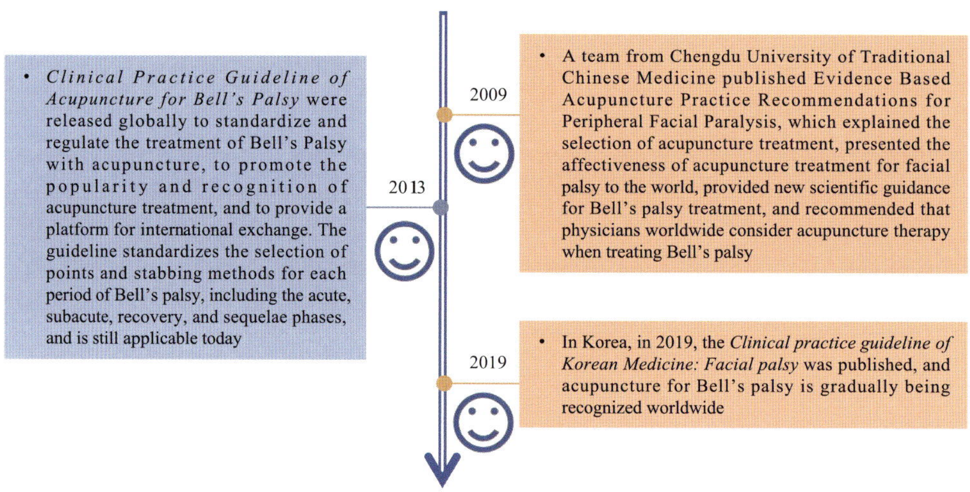

Figure 5　Summary of Clinical Guideline Recommendations for Acupuncture in the Treatment of Facial Paralysis

3. 带状疱疹

3. Herpes zoster

1）针灸治疗带状疱疹的机理

1) The mechanism of acupuncture in the treatment of herpes zoster

带状疱疹是由水痘－带状疱疹病毒感染引起的一种急性疱疹性皮肤病，发病时局部先觉皮肤灼热、疼痛，感觉过敏，继而出现皮肤潮红及簇集粟粒大小丘疹，迅速变为小水疱，附近淋巴结肿大。皮疹好发于胸、背、面、颈、腰腹部，单侧发疹，常沿皮神经分布。带状疱疹属于中医学“缠腰火丹”“蛇串疮”等范畴，主要由肝经郁热、湿热内蕴兼感邪毒所致，故以清热、利湿、解毒为主要治则[37]。本病发病过程中，由于病毒侵犯局部神经根引起神经炎症反应出现明显的神经痛，中医认为邪气入络，遂采用针灸方法通调络脉，达到通则不痛的效果[38]。

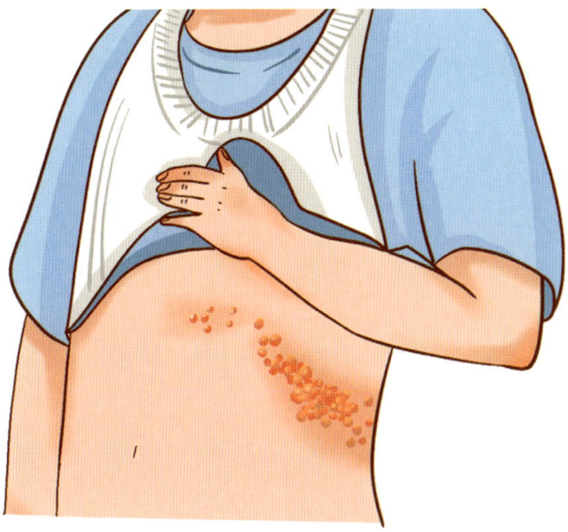

[37] 王丽华，宋丽璇，刘嘉，等．益气排毒汤治疗气虚毒滞型带状疱疹疗效观察[J]. 中华中医药学刊,2023,41(2):185-188.

[38] 刘春阳，王莒生，刘志勇．针药联合治疗带状疱疹急性期肝经郁热证52例疗效观察[J]. 中医杂志,2017,58(21):1842-1845.

Herpes zoster is an acute herpetic skin disease caused by varicella zoster virus infection, in which the skin is burning, painful and hyperesthetic, followed by skin flushing and clusters of corn grain-sized papules, which rapidly become small blisters, and the nearby lymph nodes are enlarged. The rash occurs on the chest, back, face, neck, waist and abdomen, usually on one side of the body, often distributed along the cutaneous nerve. Herpes zoster falls under the category of "snakelike sores" and "spider sores" in traditional Chinese medicine, and is etiologically and pathologically characterized by liver meridian heat, dampness and heat internalization and an attack by external pathological factors. The treatment should be focusing on clearing away heat and dampness and detoxifying the organs. During the onset of this disease, the virus invades the local nerve roots and causes the inflammatory reaction of the nerves and acute neuralgia. Traditional Chinese medicine believes this to be reflecting the evil qi entering the collaterals, so applies acupuncture to regulate and re-align the collaterals and relieve pain.

2）针灸治疗带状疱疹的临床疗效循证评价

2) Systematic evaluation of clinical effect of acupuncture on herpes zoster

（1）带状疱疹

（1）Herpes zoster

2021 年，一项纳入 21 个随机对照试验，共涉及 1577 名带状疱疹参与者的系统评价显示：与抗病毒治疗相比，针灸可使 VAS 评分降低，并减少结痂和脱痂时间，降低带状疱疹后遗神经痛（PHN）发生率[39]（见表 5）。

In 2021, a systematic review that included 21 RCTs involving a total of 1577 participants with herpes zoster showed: compared with antiviral therapy, acupuncture was associated with a reduction in VAS score, incrustation time, decrustation time, and incidence of post-herpetic neuralgia (PHN) (see table 5).

---

[39] CUI Y, WANG F, LI H, et al. Efficacy of acupuncture for herpes zoster: A systematic review and meta-analysis. wirksamkeit von akupunktur bei herpes zoster: eine systematische ü bersicht und metaanalyse [J]. Complement Med Res, 2021, 28(5): 463-472.

（2）带状疱疹后遗疼痛

（2）Post-herpetic neuralgia

2019 年，一项纳入 8 个随机对照试验，共涉及 498 名带状疱疹后遗疼痛参与者的系统评价显示：针刺有助于缓解疼痛强度，不同干预类型的亚组分析显示，电针、火针和放血拔罐对缓解疼痛强度较对照有更好的效果。针灸组的汉密尔顿焦虑量表评分（HAMA）低于对照组[40]（见表 5）。

In 2019, a systematic review that included 8 RCTs involving a total of 498 participants with post-herpetic neuralgia showed: acupuncture helped relieve pain intensity. Subgroup analysis of the different types showed that electro-acupuncture (EA), fire needling, bloodletting and cupping, and acupoint injection each relieved more pain than the controls. The Hamilton Anxiety Scale (HAMA) score was lower for the acupuncture group than for the control group (see table 5).

表 5　针灸治疗带状疱疹临床疗效循证评价证据总结表

改善指标	对照类型	纳入研究数量	纳入患者数量		WMD/SMD (or RR) (95%CI)	GRADE 证据分级
			试验组	对照组		
带状疱疹						
VAS[1]	针灸 vs 抗病毒	11	456	459	WMD: −16.13 (−19.77 to −12.49)	低等
结痂时间	针灸 vs 抗病毒	11	347	355	WMD: −1.86 (−2.38 to −1.34)	低等
脱痂时间	针灸 vs 抗病毒	5	175	183	WMD: −2.19 (−2.54 to −1.84)	低等
PHN[2] 发生率	针灸 vs 抗病毒	6	342	342	RR: 0.17 (0.10 to 0.27)	中等
带状疱疹后遗神经痛						
疼痛强度[3]	针灸[5] vs 药物	8	250	248	SMD: −1.78 (−2.36 to −1.21)	中等
HAMA[4]	针灸[6] vs 药物	2	60	60	SMD: −18.94 (−37.37 to −0.52)	低等

注：WMD，加权平均差；SMD，标准平均差；CI，置信区间；RR，风险比。1，视觉模拟量表（VAS）；2，带状疱疹后神经痛（PHN）；3，疼痛强度的变化通过 VAS、数字评定量表（NRS）、麦吉尔疼痛问卷（MPQ）、口头评定量表（VRS）以及其他几种测量疼痛的量表进行测量；4，汉密尔顿焦虑量表（HAMA）；5，电针、火针、放血拔罐和穴位注射；6，电针和电针加穴位注射。

[40] PEI W, ZWNG J, LU L, et al. Is acupuncture an effective postherpetic neuralgia treatment? A systematic review and meta-analysis [J]. J Pain Res, 2019, 12: 2155-2165.

Table 5 Summary of Evidence for the Effectiveness of Acupuncture in the Treatment of Herpes Zoster

Outcomes	Comparison	No. of Studies	No. of Patients		WMD/SMD (or RR) (95%CI)	Certainty of the Evidence (GRADE)
			T	C		
Herpes Zoster						
VAS[1]	Acupuncture vs Antiviral therapy	11	456	459	WMD: −16.13 (−19.77 to −12.49)	Low
Incrustation Time	Acupuncture vs Antiviral Therapy	11	347	355	WMD: −1.86 (−2.38 to −1.34)	Low
Decrustation Time	Acupuncture vs Antiviral Therapy	5	175	183	WMD: −2.19 (−2.54 to −1.84)	Low
Incidence of PHN[2]	Acupuncture vs Antiviral Therapy	6	342	342	RR: 0.17 (0.10 to 0.27)	Moderate
Post−herpetic Neuralgia						
Pain Intensity[3]	Acupuncture[5] vs Medicine	8	250	248	SMD: −1.78 (−2.36 to −1.21)	Moderate
HAMA[4]	Acupuncture[6] vs Medicine	2	60	60	SMD: −18.94 (−37.37 to −0.52)	Low

Note: SMD,standardized mean difference; RR, risk ratio; CI, confidence interval; T, treatment group; C, control group. 1, Visual Analog Scale (VAS); 2, Post-herpetic Neuralgia (PHN). 3, the change of pain intensity was measured by the VAS, Numerical Rating Scale (NRS), McGill Pain Questionnaire (MPQ), Verbal Rating Scale (VRS) as well as several other scales for measuring pain; 4, Hamilton Anxiety Scale (HAMA); 5, electro-acupuncture, fire needling, bloodletting and cupping, and acupoint injection; 6, electro-acupuncture, and electro-acupuncture plus acupoint injection.

3）针灸治疗带状疱疹循证指南推荐

3) Clinical guideline recommendations for acupuncture in the treatment of herpes zoster

2013 年，广安门团队基于当时已有的临床研究证据和专家经验，制定了针灸治疗带状疱疹的指南，指南中详细描述了带状疱疹不同时期的针刺选穴、针刺手法

（火针、针刺放血等）、疗程、注意事项等，为带状疱疹的针灸治疗提供了借鉴价值[41]。针灸治疗带状疱疹临床指南推荐意见总结见图 6。

In 2013, the team from Guang'anmen hospital developed a guideline for the treatment of herpes zoster with acupuncture based on the clinical research evidence available and the experience of experts. The guideline described in detail the selection of points for acupuncture, acupuncture maneuvers (fire acupuncture, needle bloodletting, etc.), course of treatment, and precautions to be taken at different periods of herpes zoster, which provided guidance for the treatment of herpes zoster with acupuncture. Summary of clinical guideline recommendations for acupuncture in the treatment of herpes zoster is shown in figure 6.

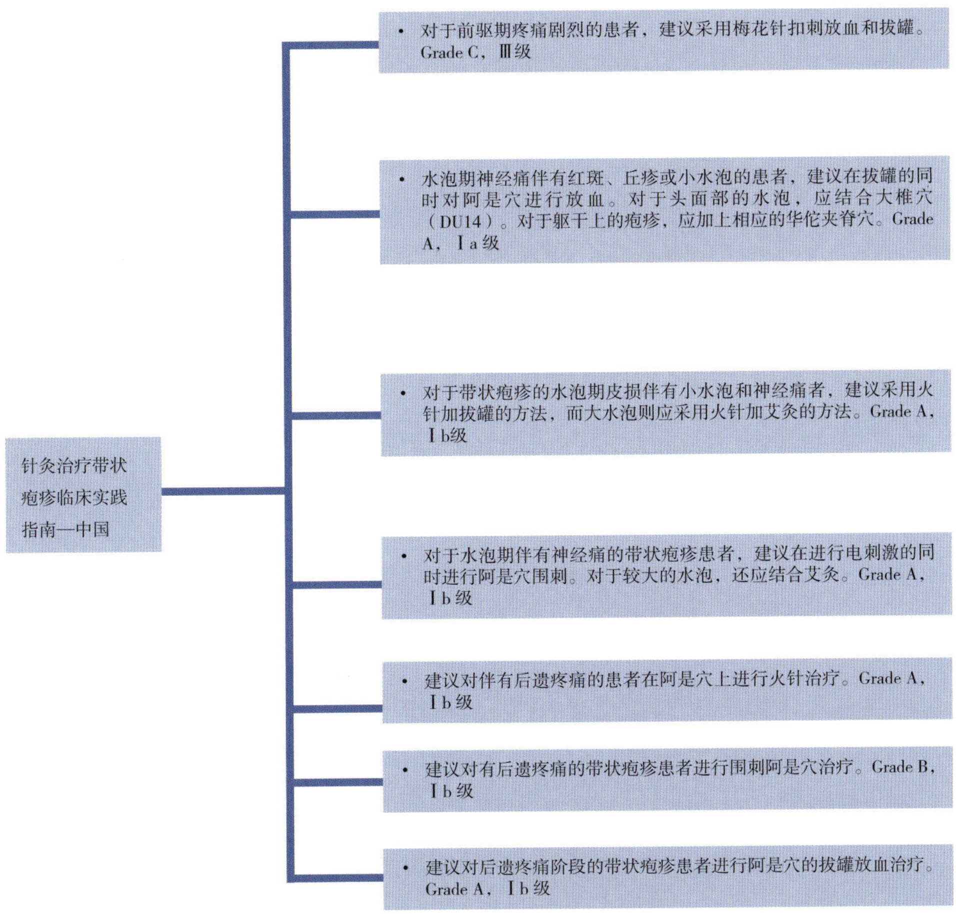

图 6　针灸治疗带状疱疹临床指南推荐意见总结

[41] LIU ZS, PENG WN, LIU BY, et al. Clinical practice guideline of acupuncture for herpes zoster [J]. Chin J Integr Med, 2013, 19(1): 58-67.

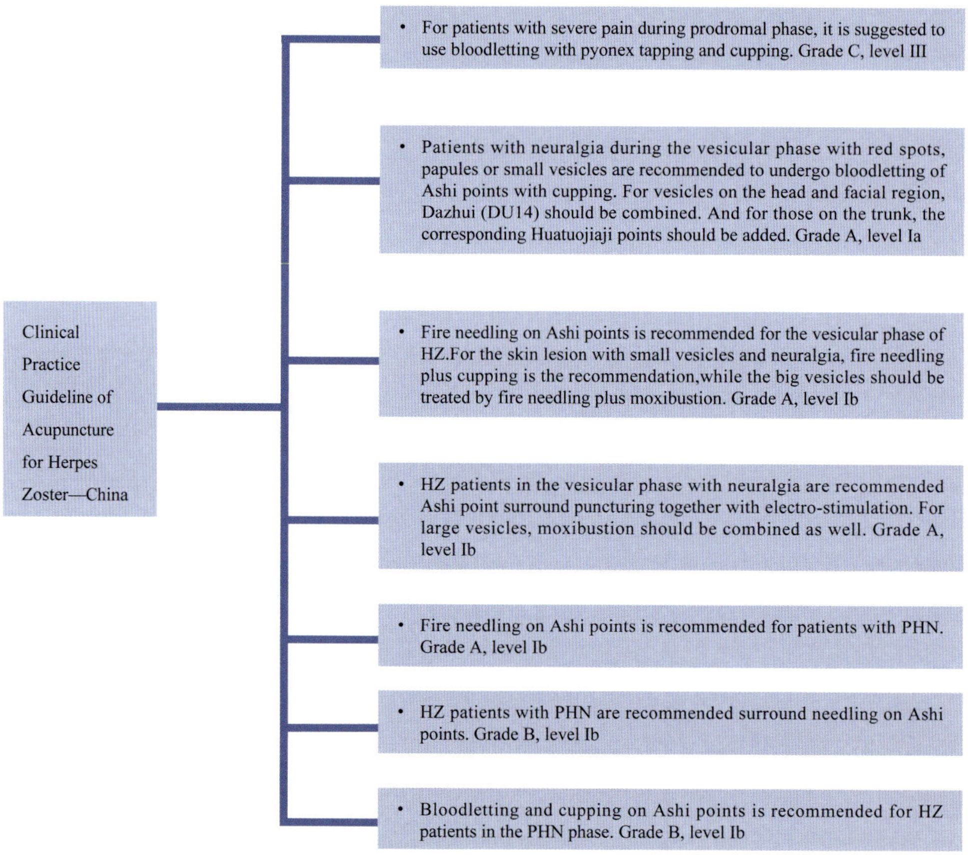

Figure 6 Summary of Clinical Guideline Recommendations for Acupuncture in the Treatment of Herpes Zoster

4. 失眠

4. Insomnia

1）针灸治疗失眠的机理

1) The mechanism of acupuncture in the treatment of insomnia

失眠是指尽管有合适的睡眠机会和睡眠环境，患者依然对睡眠时间和（或）质量不满足并影响日间社会功能的主观体验，表现为入睡困难、睡眠维持障碍、早醒、睡眠质量下降和总睡眠时间减少，同时伴有日间功能障碍[42]。失眠属于中医学“不寐”的范畴，多由脏腑阴阳失调所致，以心神失养为主要病机。针灸通过刺激人体的额和顶区的神经，作用于下丘脑背部，调节睡眠—觉醒功能，还可改变头部血液循环，激活神经元，起到治疗失眠的目的[43]。

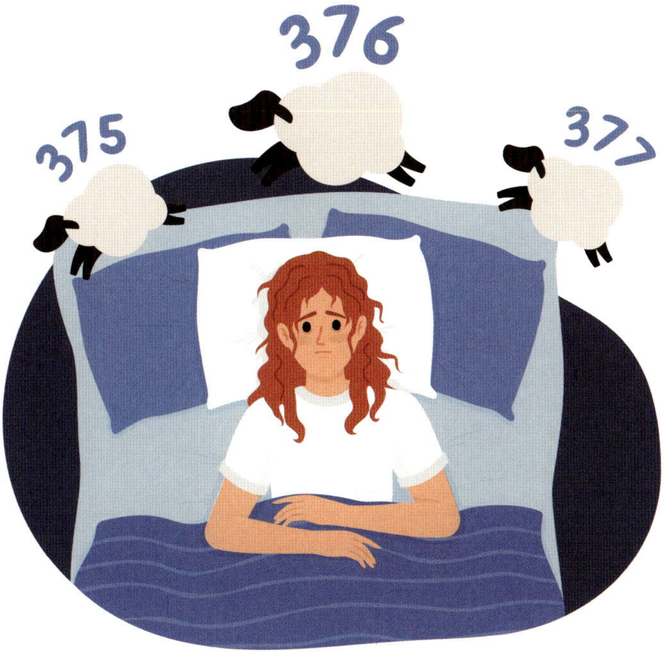

Insomnia serves as a subjective experience that patients are still dissatisfied with the length and/or quality of sleep, which affects their daytime social functioning despite appropriate sleep opportunities and environment, manifested by difficulty in falling and remaining asleep, waking early, decreased sleep quality and total sleep time, accompanied by daytime dysfunction. Insomnia is defined as “difficulty sleeping” in traditional Chinese medicine, which is mostly caused by the imbalance of yin and yang in the internal organs, with the loss of nourishment of the mind and spirit as the main pathological cause. Acupuncture can stimulate the nerves in the frontal and parietal regions of the human body, act on the back of the hypothalamus, and regulate sleep-wakefulness function, while also changing the blood circulation of the head and activating neurons, thereby treating insomnia.

[42] 陆静珏，许文杰．老年慢性失眠慢病管理指南 [J]. 中西医结合研究 ,2023,15(5):311-324.

[43] 李虎成，高齐，李永宏．针刺督脉穴治疗失眠的疗效观察及对患者血清神经递质水平的影响 [J]. 上海针灸杂志 ,2023,42(10):1030-1035.

2）针灸治疗失眠临床疗效循证评价
2) Systematic evaluation of clinical effect of acupuncture on insomnia

（1）原发性失眠
（1）Primary insomnia

2019 年，一项纳入 73 个随机对照试验，共涉及 5533 名原发性失眠参与者的系统评价显示：针灸治疗与空白对照或假针灸对比，或针灸加艾司唑仑与单用艾司唑仑对比，针灸在降低匹兹堡睡眠质量指数（Pittsburgh sleep quality index, PSQI）总分方面更有效。针灸对 PSQI 总分的降低效果优于艾司唑仑，且下降程度与艾司唑仑剂量成反比。在阿森斯失眠量表（Athens insomnia scale, AIS）评分和 SPIEGEL 评分，针灸比苯二氮卓类药物更能改善患者的整体睡眠质量。在安全性方面，针灸的不良事件约为西药组的四分之一[44]（见表 6）。

In 2019, a systematic review that included a total of 73 RCTs involving 5533 primary insomnia participants were showed: For comparison of acupuncture with no treatment, sham acupuncture, or acupuncture plus estazolam compared with estazolam alone, acupuncture appeared to be more effective on decreasing Pittsburgh Sleep Quality Index (PSQI) total scores. Acupuncture showed better effect on decreasing the PSQI total scores than estazolam, and the degree of decline was inversely proportional to the dose of estazolam. The pooled results also showed that acupuncture could improve patients' overall quality of sleep than benzodiazepines on Athens Insomnia Scale (AIS) scale and SPIEGEL scale. The results showed that the incidence of adverse events in acupuncture group was about a quarter of the western medicine group (see table 6).

（2）卒中后失眠
（2）Post-stroke insomnia

2023 年，一项纳入 41 个随机对照试验，共涉及 3233 名卒中后失眠参与者的系统评价显示：针灸在改善 PSQI 总分、提高睡眠效率和总睡眠时间方面均优于对照组（CG）。在针灸加 CG 与 CG 的比较中，也观察到了改善 PSQI 总分、减少睡眠潜伏期和增加总睡眠时间的良好结果。在长期疗效和安全性方面，针灸的疗效具有长期性

[44] CAO HJ, YU ML, WANG LQ, et al. Acupuncture for primary insomnia: an updated systematic review of randomized controlled trials [J]. J Altern Complement Med, 2019, 25(5): 451-474.

和稳健性，但由于安全性资料有限，无法得出可靠的安全性结论[45]（详见表 6）。

In 2023, a systematic review that included a total of 41 RCTs involving 3233 post-stroke insomnia participants were analyzed showed: acupuncture was superior to control group (CG) in improving PSQI total score, increasing sleep efficiency and total sleep time. The favorable results in improving PSQI total score, reduced sleep latency and increased total sleep time were also observed in comparisons of acupuncture plus CG vs CG. As of long-term efficacy and safety, the effects of acupuncture were long-term and robustness, however, due to limited safety information, reliable safety conclusions cannot be drawn (see table 6).

表 6　针灸治疗失眠临床疗效循证评价证据总结表

改善指标	对照类型	纳入研究数量	纳入患者数量		SMD/MD（或 RR）(95%CI)	GRADE 证据分级
			试验组	对照组		
原发性失眠						
PSQI[1]	针灸 vs 空白对照	2	105		MD: −5.58 (−6.85 to −4.31)	极低等
	针灸 vs 苯二氮䓬类药物	32	2452		MD: −1.73 (−2.11 to −1.35)	极低等
	针灸 vs 非苯二氮䓬类药物	9	643		MD: −0.94 (−1.55 to −0.33)	极低等
	针灸 + 艾司唑仑 vs 艾司唑仑	4	253		MD: −3.17 (−4.74 to −1.61)	低等
SPIEGEL[2]	针灸 vs 苯二氮䓬类药物	5	326		MD: −2.86 (−3.54 to −2.18)	极低等
AIS3	针灸 vs 苯二氮䓬类药物	3	180		MD: −1.64 (−2.40 to −0.89)	极低等
不良事件	针灸 vs 西药	11	914		RR: 0.23 (0.11 to 0.48)	低等
卒中后失眠						
PSQI	针灸 vs 药物	26	1083	889	SMD: −1.03 (−1.32 to −0.74)	极低等
	针灸 + 药物 vs 药物	15	629	602	SMD: −1.26 (−1.57 to −0.94)	极低等

[45] SHI M, JI Z, SUN T, et al. Efficacy and safety of acupuncture on sleep quality for post-stroke insomnia: A systematic review and meta-analysis [J]. Front Neurol. 2023, 14: 1164604.

续表

改善指标	对照类型	纳入研究数量	纳入患者数量		SMD/MD（或 RR）(95%CI)	GRADE 证据分级
			试验组	对照组		
长期疗效[4]	针灸 vs 药物[6]	6	283	214	SMD: −0.88 (−1.30 to −0.46)	低等
	针灸 vs 药物[7]	4	204	130	SMD: −1.29 (−2.12 to −0.46)	极低等
	针灸 + 药物 vs 药物	2	67	67	SMD: −1.20 (−1.99 to −0.42)	极低等
总睡眠时间[5]	针灸 vs 药物	2	79	77	SMD: 0.54 (0.22 to 0.86)	低等
	针灸 + 药物 vs 药物	3	109	107	SMD: 1.84 (0.31 to 3.38)	低等
睡眠有效率[5]	针灸 vs 药物	3	169	168	SMD: 0.65 (0.37 to 0.92)	低等
睡眠潜伏期[5]	针灸 + 药物 vs 药物	2	120	119	SMD: −0.73 (−1.15 to −0.31)	极低等

注：SMD，标准平均差；MD，平均差；RR，风险比。1，匹兹堡睡眠质量指数（PSQI）由 7 个因子的 19 个项目组成，总分范围为 0~21 分；2，SPIEGEL 总分范围为 0 ～ 30 分；3，雅典失眠量表（AIS）总分范围为 0 ～ 24 分；4，使用随访数据评估长期效果；5，通过多导睡眠图（PSG）测量客观睡眠数据，如睡眠开始潜伏期、睡眠效率和总睡眠时间；6，随访时间（治疗后第一个月）；7，随访时间（治疗后第三个月）。

Table 6 Summary of Evidence for the Effectiveness of Acupuncture in the Treatment of Insomnia

Outcomes	Comparison	No. of Studies	No. of Patients		SMD/MD (or RR) (95%CI)	Certainty of the Evidence (GRADE)
			T	C		
Primary Insomnia						
PSQI[1]	Acupuncture vs No Treatment	2	105		MD: −5.58 (−6.85 to −4.31)	Very Low
	Acupuncture vs Benzodiazepines	32	2452		MD: −1.73 (−2.11 to −1.35)	Very Low
	Acupuncture vs Nonbenzodiazepines	9	643		MD: −0.94 (−1.55 to −0.33)	Very Low
	Acupuncture Plus Estazolam vs Estazolam	4	253		MD: −3.17 (−4.74 to −1.61)	Low

continued table 6

Outcomes	Comparison	No. of Studies	No. of Patients		SMD/MD (or RR) (95%CI)	Certainty of the Evidence (GRADE)
			T	C		
SPIEGEL[2]	Acupuncture vs benzodiazepines	5	326		MD: −2.86 (−3.54 to −2.18)	Very Low
AIS[3]	Acupuncture vs benzodiazepines	3	180		MD: −1.64 (−2.40 to −0.89)	Very Low
Adverse Event	Acupuncture vs West Medicine	11	914		RR: 0.23 (0.11 to 0.48)	Low
Post-stroke Insomnia						
PSQI	Acupuncture vs Medicine	26	1083	889	SMD: −1.03 (−1.32 to −0.74)	Very Low
	Acupuncture Plus Medicine vs Medicine	15	629	602	SMD: −1.26 (−1.57 to −0.94)	Very Low
Long-term Efficacy[4]	Acupuncture vs Medicine[6]	6	283	214	SMD: −0.88 (−1.30 to −0.46)	Low
	Acupuncture vs Medicine[7]	4	204	130	SMD: −1.29 (−2.12 to −0.46)	Very Low
	Acupuncture Plus Medicine vs Medicine	2	67	67	SMD: −1.20 (−1.99 to −0.42)	Very Low
Total Sleep Time[5]	Acupuncture vs Medicine	2	79	77	SMD: 0.54 (0.22 to 0.86)	Low
	Acupuncture Plus Medicine vs Medicine	3	109	107	SMD: 1.84 (0.31 to 3.38)	Low
Sleep Efficiency[5]	Acupuncture vs Medicine	3	169	168	SMD: 0.65 (0.37 to 0.92)	Low
Sleep Latency[5]	Acupuncture Plus Medicine vs Medicine	2	120	119	SMD: −0.73 (−1.15 to −0.31)	Very Low

Note: SMD, standardized mean difference; MD, mean difference; CI, confidence interval; T, treatment group; C, control group. 1, Pittsburgh Sleep Quality Index (PSQI) consists of 19 items in 7 factors and the total scores range from 0 to 21; 2, the total scores of SPIEGEL range from 0 to 30; 3, the total scores of Athens Insomnia Scale (AIS) range from 0 to 24; 4, using data from follow-up visits to evaluate the long-term effects; 5, objective sleep data was measured by polysomnography (PSG), such as sleep onset latency, sleep efficiency and total sleep time; 6, follow-up time (first month after treatment). 7, follow-up time (third month after treatment).

3）针灸治疗失眠循证指南推荐

3) Clinical guideline recommendations for acupuncture in the treatment of insomnia

由于没有方法学质量足够高的研究支持针灸用于失眠的治疗，在 2009 年西班牙 [46]、2016 年美国 [47] 和 2017 年欧洲 [48] 发布的失眠治疗相关指南中，均未对针

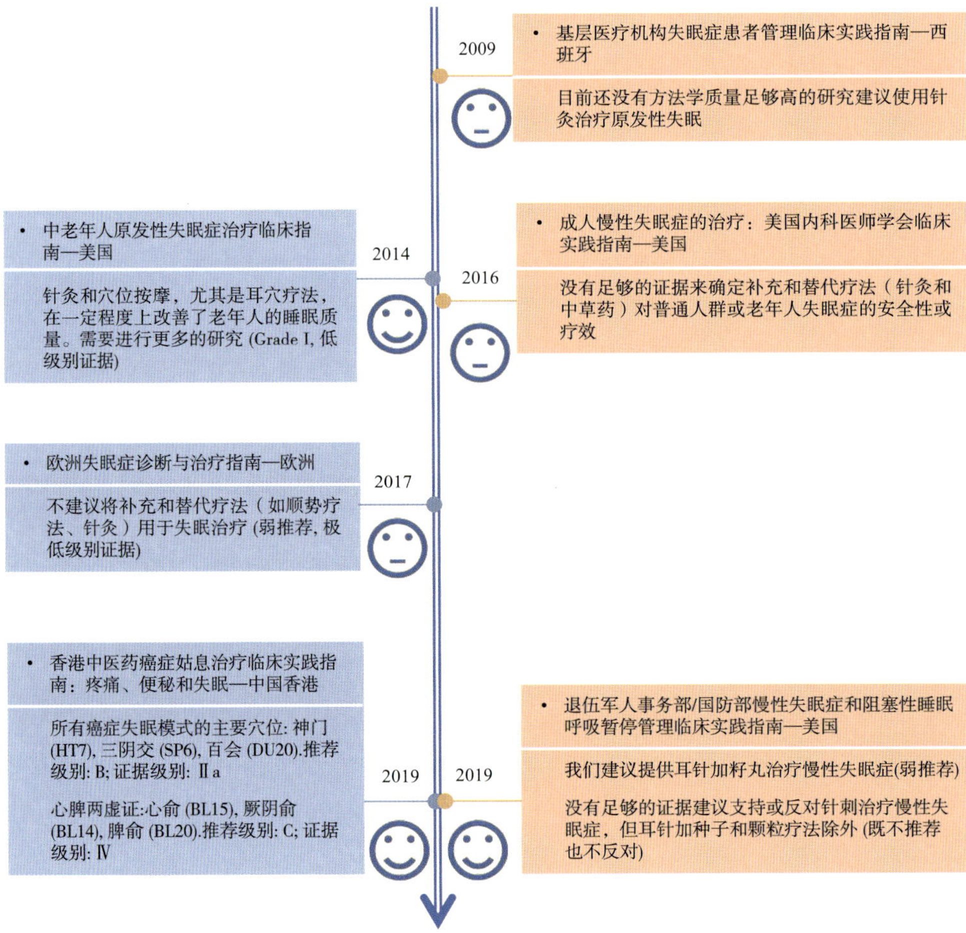

图 7　针灸治疗失眠临床指南推荐意见总结

[46] Ministry of Science and Innovation. Clinical practice guidelines for the management of patients with insomnia in primary care [M]. Ministry of Science and Innovation, 2009.

[47] QASEEM A, KANSAGARA D, FORCIEA MA, et al. Management of chronic insomnia disorder in adults: a clinical practice guideline from the American College of Physicians [J]. Ann Intern Med, 2016, 165(2): 125-133.

[48] RIEMANN D, BAG LIONI BASSETTI C, Bassetti C, et al. European guideline for the diagnosis and treatment of insomnia [J]. J Sleep Res, 2017, 26(6): 675-700.

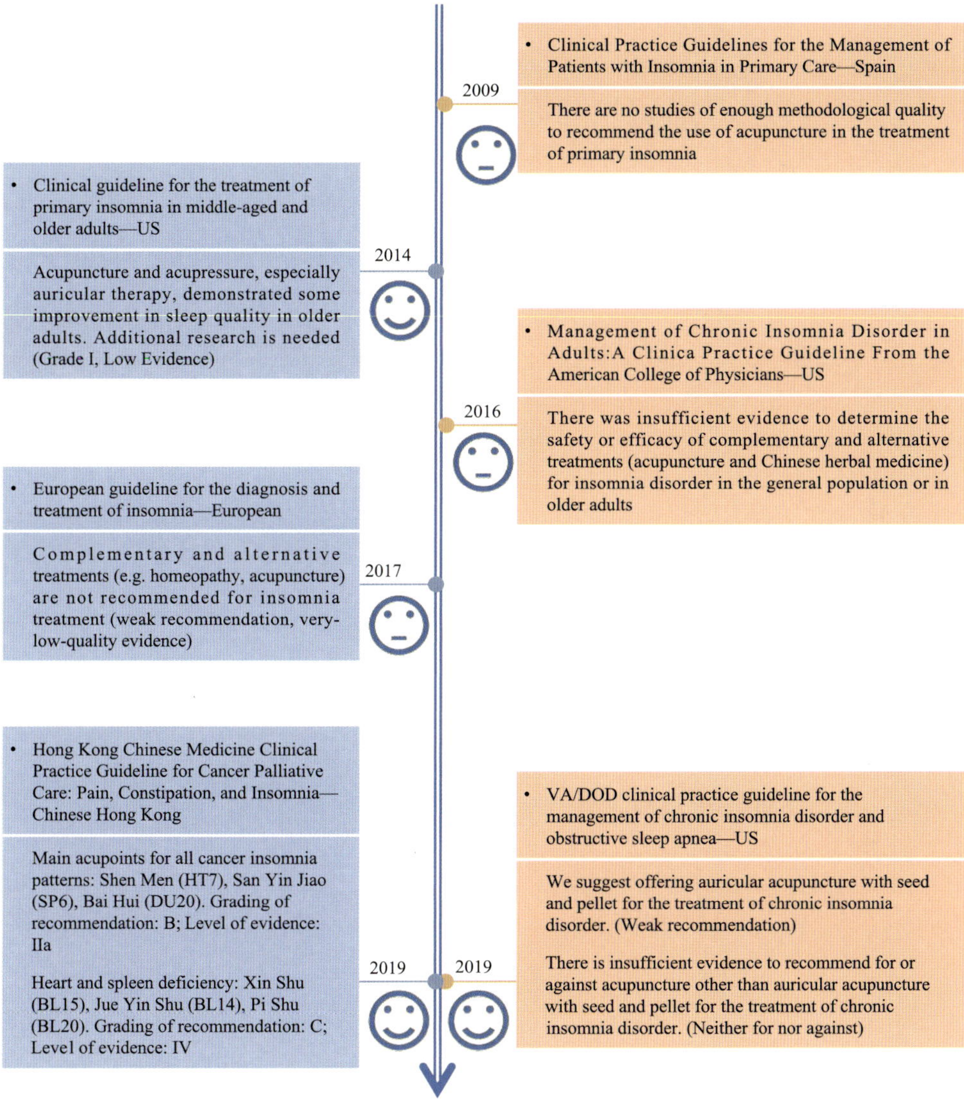

Figure 7　Summary of Clinical Guideline Recommendations for Acupuncture in the Treatment of Insomnia

灸做出明确推荐。在 2014 年美国发布的中老年人原发性失眠治疗的指南中，一定程度上推荐了针灸和穴位按摩，尤其是耳穴疗法用于改善了老年人的睡眠质量，但需要进行更多的研究 [49]。随后，美国在 2019 年治疗慢性失眠症的指南中推荐采用

[49] University of Texas at Austin School of Nursing, Family Nurse Practitioner Program. Clinical guideline for the treatment of primary insomnia in middle-aged and older adults [M]. Austin (TX) University of Texas at Austin, School of Nursing, 2014, 28.

耳穴疗法[50]。同年，在中国香港发布的癌症姑息疗法的指南中，推荐了针灸用于癌症引起的失眠[51]。针灸治疗失眠临床指南推荐意见总结见图7。

Due to the absence of studies of sufficiently high methodological quality to support the use of acupuncture for the treatment of insomnia, acupuncture was not recommended in the guidelines related to the treatment of insomnia published in Spain in 2009, in the United States (US) in 2016, and in Europe in 2017. In the guidelines for the treatment of primary insomnia in middle-aged and older adults released in the US in 2014, acupuncture and acupressure, especially auricular acupressure, were recommended to some extent for improving the quality of sleep in older adults, but more research was needed. Afterwards, auricular acupressure was also recommended in the US in the 2019 guideline for the treatment of chronic insomnia. In the same year, acupuncture was recommended for cancer-induced insomnia in guidelines for palliative care for cancer released in Chinese Hong Kong. Summary of clinical guideline recommendations for acupuncture in the treatment of insomnia is shown in figure 7.

5. 下背部疼痛

5. Low back pain

1）针灸治疗下背部疼痛的机理

1) The mechanism of acupuncture in the treatment of low back pain

中医学认为下背部疼痛病机以气血不畅，经脉瘀阻为主。针灸作用于人体的经络系统，能通调周身气血、调阴阳、扶正祛邪、疏通经络，达到瘀去新生，通则不痛的效果[52]。而现代机制研究[53]则认为针灸通过降低腰部组织神经末梢的兴奋性，促进紧张痉挛的肌肉松弛，扩张周围血管以改变局部微循环缺血缺氧的病理状态，

[50] Office of Quality, Safety and Value, VA, Washington DC; Office of Evidence Based Practice, U.S. Army Medical Command. VA/DOD clinical practice guideline for the management of chronic insomnia disorder and obstructive sleep apnea [M]. Office of Quality, Safety and Value, VA, Washington DC; Office of Evidence Based Practice, U.S. Army Medical Command, 2019.

[51] LAM WC, ZHONG L, LIU Y, et al. Hong Kong Chinese medicine clinical practice guideline for cancer palliative care: pain, constipation, and insomnia [J]. Evid Based Complement Alternat Med, 2019: 1038206.

[52] 刘伟，江蓉星，陈子锴，等．非特异性下腰痛病因与治疗方案分析 [J]. 中医临床研究 ,2016,8(5):146-148.

[53] LEE JH, CHOI, TY, LEE, MS, et al. Acupuncture for acute low back pain: a systematic review [J]. Clin J Pain, 2013, 29(2): 172-185.

消除局部组织的炎症和水肿，从而恢复腰部正常的生物力学平衡状态，减轻下背部疼痛患者的症状，改善腰部的功能活动。

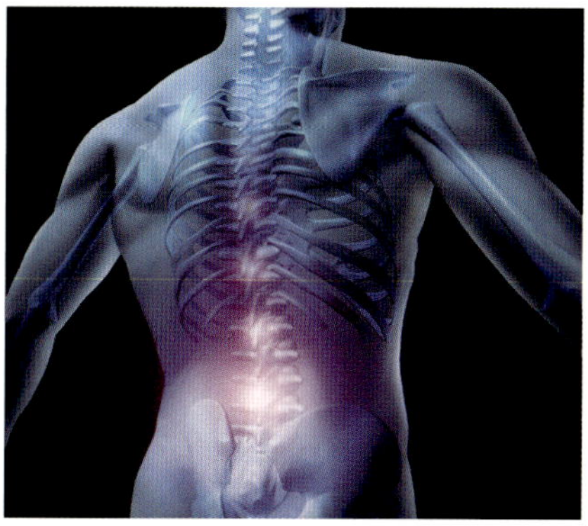

Traditional Chinese medicine believes that the pathogenesis of low back pain is mainly from unsmoothed qi and blood and obstructed meridians. Acupuncture, acting on the human body's meridian system, can regulate the body's qi and blood, adjust the yin and yang, support the inner strength of the body and unblock the meridians. The outcome is that dispel stasis to unlock collaterals and dissipate pains. Modern medicine research holds that acupuncture reduces the excitability of the lumbar tissue nerve endings, relaxes muscle tension and spasm and dilates peripheral blood vessels to change the pathological state of local microcirculation ischemia and hypoxia, to eliminate the inflammation and edema of the local tissues. That is helpful to restore the normal biomechanical equilibrium of the waist area, reducing the symptoms of the patients with pain in the low back, and improving the functionalities.

2）针灸治疗下背部疼痛临床疗效循证评价

2) Systematic evaluation of clinical effect of acupuncture on low back pain

2020 年，一项基于 33 个随机对照试验，涉及 8270 名下背部疼痛患者的 Cochrane 系统评价显示[54]，短期内，针灸在缓解疼痛或改善患者生活质量方面可能并不比安慰针灸更有临床意义的作用，而且在短期内，针灸可能并不比安慰干预更能改善背部功能。但针灸在短期内改善疼痛和功能方面比不治疗更有效。以常规治疗作为对照的试验表明，针灸在临床上可能不会减轻疼痛，但可以立即改善身体

[54] MU J, FURLAN AD, LAM WY, et al. Acupuncture for chronic nonspecific low back pain [J]. Cochrane Database Syst Rev, 2020, 12(12): CD013814.

功能，并在短期内改善身体方面的生活质量（见表 7）。

In 2020, A Cochrane systematic review included 33 RCTs with 8270 participants with low back pain showed: acupuncture might not play a more clinically meaningful role than sham intervention in relieving pain immediately after treatment or in improving patients' quality of life in the short term, and acupuncture possibly did not improve back function compared to sham intervention in the immediate term. However, acupuncture was more effective than no treatment in improving pain and function in the immediate term. Trials with usual care as the control showed acupuncture might not reduce pain clinically, but the therapy might improve function immediately after sessions as well as physical but not mental quality of life in the short term (see table 7).

表 7　针灸治疗下背部疼痛临床疗效循证评价证据总结表

改善指标	对照类型	纳入研究数量	纳入患者数量		SMD（或 MD）(95%CI)	GRADE 证据分级
			试验组	对照组		
疼痛强度（VAS）[1]	针灸 vs 假干预	7	735	668	MD: −9.22 (−13.82 to −4.61)	低等
	针灸 vs 无治疗	4	216	150	MD: −20.32 (−24.50 to −16.14)	中等
	针灸 vs 常规治疗	5	531	523	MD: −10.26(−17.11 to −3.40)	低等
背部特定功能状态[2]	针灸 vs 假干预	5	769	712	SMD: −0.16(−0.38 to 0.06)	极低等
	针灸 vs 无治疗	5	1566	1394	SMD: −0.53(−0.73 to −0.34)	中等
	针灸 vs 常规治疗	5	703	678	SMD: −0.47(−0.77 to −0.17)	低等
生活质量[3]（QoL）	针灸 vs 假干预	3	568	500	SMD: 0.24(0.03 to 0.45)	低等
	针灸 vs 常规治疗 SF−12 生理	1	370	361	MD: 4.20(2.82 to 5.58)	中等
	针灸 vs 常规治疗 SF−12 精	1	370	361	MD: 1.90(0.25 to 3.55)	中等

注：SMD，标准平均差；MD，平均差；CI，置信区间。1，视觉模拟评分（VAS，0 ～ 100；0 = 无痛，100 = 最严重的痛）。随访时间：治疗结束后立即随访，或在治疗结束后 7 天内随访。2，HFAQl（平山功能评估量表）得分（0 ～ 100；0 = 残疾，100 = 完全功能）。随访时间：治疗结束后立即随访，或在治疗结束后 7 天内随访。3，SF−12 量表评分（0 至 100；0 = 较差的生活质量，100 = 较高的生活质量）。随访时间：短期随访，8 天至 3 个月。

Table 7 Summary of Evidence for the Effectiveness of Acupuncture in the Treatment of Chronic Nonspecific Low Back Pain

Outcomes	Comparison		No. of studies	No. of patients		MD(95%CI)	Certainty of the evidence (GRADE)
				T	C		
Pain Intensity[1] (VAS)	Acupuncture vs Sham Intervention		7	735	668	MD: −9.22 (−13.82 to −4.61)	Low
	Acupuncture vs No Treatment		4	216	150	MD: −20.32 (−24.50 to −16.14)	Moderate
	Acupuncture vs Usual Care		5	531	523	MD: −10.26 (−17.11 to −3.40)	Low
Back-specific Functional Status[2]	Acupuncture vs Sham Intervention		5	769	712	SMD: −0.16 (−0.38 to 0.06)	Very Low
	Acupuncture vs No Treatment		5	1566	1394	SMD: −0.53 (−0.73 to −0.34)	Moderate
	Acupuncture vs Usual Care		5	703	678	SMD: −0.47 (−0.77 to −0.17)	Low
Quality of Life (QoL)[3]	Acupuncture vs Sham Intervention		3	568	500	SMD: 0.24 (0.03 to 0.45)	Low
	Acupuncture vs Usual Care	SF-12 Physical	1	370	361	MD: 4.20 (2.82 to 5.58)	Moderate
		SF-12 Mental	1	370	361	MD: 1.90 (0.25 to 3.55)	Moderate

Note: 1, VAS (0 ～ 100; 0 = no pain, 100 = worst pain). Follow-up: immediately after; < 7 days after the end of the sessions. 2,HFAQ (hirayama functionality assessment questionnaire)(0 ～ 100; 0 = disabled, 100 = full function) Follow-up: immediately after; < 7 days after the end of the sessions. 3, SF-12 (0 ～ 100; 0 = poor QoL, 100 = high QoL). Follow-up: short term; 8 days to 3 months.

3）针灸治疗下背部疼痛循证指南推荐

3) Clinical guideline recommendations for acupuncture in the treatment of low back pain

鉴于针灸在治疗下背部疼痛的潜在优势，1994 年，美国医疗保健政策研究所在 *Acute low back problems in adults: assessment and treatment* 中提及针灸治疗[55]，但因证据不足，没有将此疗法推荐给急性下背部疼痛成年患者。随着证明针灸治疗下背部疼痛相关研究不断增加，2007 年，美国医师学会和美国疼痛学会对针灸治

[55] Agency for Health Care Policy and Research. Acute low back problems in adults: assessment and treatment [J]. Am Fam Physician, 1995, 51: 469-484.

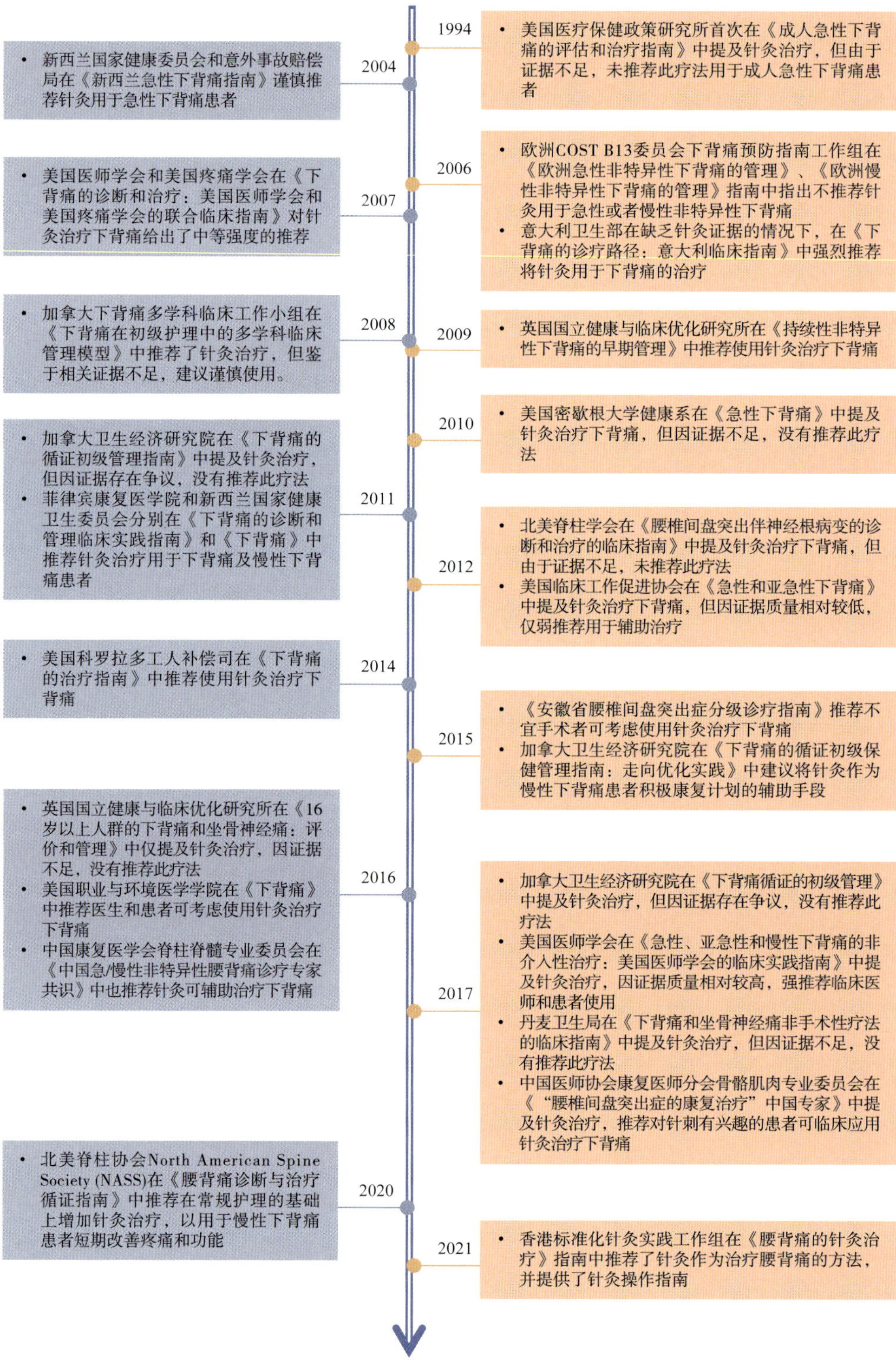

图 8　针灸治疗下背部疼痛临床指南推荐意见总结

1994

- Acupuncture was first introduced in the Guidelines for Acute Low Back Pain in Adults: Assessment and Treatment by the Agency for Health Care Policy and Research in the United States, but it was not recommended for adults with acute low back pain due to insufficient evidence

2004

- The National Health Council of New Zealand and the Accident Compensation Corporation cautiously recommended acupuncture for patients with acute low back pain in the *New Zealand Guide for Acute Low Back Pain*

2006

- The European COST B13 Working Group on *Guidelines for the Management of Acute Non-Specific Low Back Pain and Guidelines for the Management of Chronic Non-Specific Low Back Pain* did not recommend acupuncture for acute or chronic nonspecific lower back pain
- The Italian Ministry of Health strongly recommended acupuncture for the treatment of low back pain in the *Pathway of Diagnosis and Treatment: Clinical Guidelines for Low Back Pain*, despite insufficient acupuncture evidence

2007

- The American College of Physicians and the American Pain Society gave acupuncture treatment for low back pain a moderate recommendation in *Diagnosis and Treatment of Low Back Pain: A Joint Clinical Practice Guideline from the American College of Physicians and the American Pain Society*

2008

- The Canadian Multidisciplinary Low Back Pain Clinical Working Group recommended acupuncture treatment in *Multidisciplinary Clinical Management Model of Low Back Pain in Primary* Care, but cautioned against its use due to insufficient evidence

2009

- The UK National Institute for Health and Clinical Excellence recommended the use of acupuncture for the treatment of low back pain in the NICE *guideline on Early Management of Persistent Non-Specific Low Back Pain*

2010

- University of Michigan Health System made statement of acupuncture for the treatment of low back pain in *Acute Low Back pain*, but did not recommend this treatment due to insufficient evidence.

2011

- The Canadian Institute of Health Economics made statement of acupuncture in *Guidelines for the Evidence-Informed Primary Care Management of Low Back Pain*, but did not recommend it due to conflicting evidence
  The Philippine Academy of Rehabilitation Medicine and National Health Committee recommended acupuncture for low back pain in *Low Back Pain Management Guideline* and *Low Back Pain* respectively

2012

- The North American Spine Society mentioned acupuncture treatment for low back pain in the Clinical Guidelines for the *Diagnosis and Treatment of Lumbar Disc Herniation with Radiculopathy*, but due to insufficient evidence, did not recommend this therapy
- The American Association for the Advancement of Clinical Work made statement of acupuncture in *Acute and subacute Lower back pain*, due to the relatively low quality of evidence, it was only weakly recommended for the treatment of low back pain as adjuvant treatment.

2014

- The Colorado Division of Workers' Compensation recommended acupuncture for the treatment of lower back pain in the *Guidelines for Treatment of Low Back Pain.*

2015

- The *Grading and Treatment Guidelines for Lumbar Disc Herniation in Anhui Province recommended that non-surgical candidates may consider acupuncture for the treatment of low back pain.*
- The Canadian Institute for Health Economics recommended acupuncture as an adjunctive treatment for active rehabilitation plans for patients with chronic low back pain in the *Evidence-based Primary Health Care Management Guidelines for Low Back Pain: Towards Optimized Practice.*

2016

- The UK National Institute for Health and Clinical Excellence (NICE) made statement of acupuncture in *Low Back pain and Sciatica in people over 16 years of age: Evaluation and Management*, but did not recommend it due to insufficient evidence.
- The American College of Occupational and Environmental Medicine recommended acupuncture to treat lower back pain in *Lower Back Pain*
- Chinese Rehabilitation Medical Association spinal cord professional committee also recommended acupuncture as an auxiliary treatment for low back pain in the *Expert Consensus on Diagnosis and Treatment of Acute/Chronic Non-specific Low Back Pain in China.*

2017

- The Canadian Institute of Health Economics mentioned acupuncture in the *Guidelines for the Evidence- Informed Primary Care Management of Low Back Pain*, but did not recommend it due to conflicting evidence.
- The American College of Physicians mentioned acupuncture in the *Noninvasive Treatments for Acute, Subacute, and Chronic Low Back Pain: A Clinical Practice Guideline from the American College of Physicians*, which strongly recommends its use by clinicians and patients due to the relatively high quality of evidence
- The Danish Health Authority mentioned acupuncture in the Clinical *Guidelines for Non-Surgical Therapy for Low Back Pain and Sciatica*, but did not recommend it due to insufficient evidence
- The Skeletal muscle Professional Committee of the Rehabilitation Physician Branch of the Chinese Medical Doctor Association mentioned acupuncture in the Chinese Expert Consensus on Rehabilitation Treatment of Lumbar Disc Herniation, recommending that patients who are interested in acupuncture can use acupuncture to treat lower back pain

2020

- North American Spine Society (NASS) stated that in patients with chronic low back pain, addition of acupuncture to usual care is recommended for short-term improvement of pain and function, in the *Evidence-based Clinical Guideline for the Diagnosis and Treatment of Low Back Pain*

2021

- The Hong Kong Taskforce of Standardized Acupuncture Practice recommended acupuncture for lower back pain in their guidelines titled Acupuncture for *Lower Back Pain*, and provided a practice guide for acupuncture

Figure 8 Summary of Clinical Guideline Recommendations for Acupuncture in the Treatment of Low Back Pain

疗下背部疼痛给出了中等强度的推荐[56,57]。此外，在很多其他国家如新西兰、意大利、英国、加拿大、菲律宾也均在指南中给出了相应的推荐。针灸治疗下背部疼痛临床指南推荐意见总结见图 8。

In view of the potential advantages of acupuncture in the treatment of low back pain, the Agency for Health Care Policy and Research in the United States first made statement of acupuncture in *Guidelines for Acute low back in adults: assessment and treatment* in 1994, but did not recommend acupuncture for adult patients with acute Low back pain due to insufficient evidence. In 2007, the American College of Physicians and the American Pain Society made a moderate recommendation of acupuncture for Low back pain, following a growing number of studies demonstrating the advantages of acupuncture for Low back pain. In addition, many other countries such as New Zealand, Italy, the United Kingdom, Canada, the Philippines have also made positive recommendations of acupuncture in their guidelines.Summary of clinical guideline recommendations for acupuncture in the treatment of low back pain is shown in figure 8.

6. 偏头痛
6. Migraine

1）针灸治疗偏头痛的机理
1) The mechanism of acupuncture in the treatment of migraine

偏头痛是一种常见的原发性头痛，以单侧或双侧搏动性疼痛为主，部分人还会伴有恶心、呕吐、烦躁不安等症状。偏头痛属于中医“头痛”范畴，其病机主要与“风、痰、瘀、热、虚”相关，在其相互影响下最终导致瘀血阻滞经络，不通而痛，因此中医临床诊治偏头痛的关键在于通经活络[58]。其中，针灸治疗能有效减轻患者的痛苦，改善患者的生活质量，且操作简单，不良反应少，因此在临床上得到了广泛的应用。

[56] BOSWELL MV, TRESCOT AM, Datta S, et al. Interventional techniques: evidence-based practice guidelines in the management of chronic spinal pain [J]. Pain Physician, 2007, 10(1): 7-111.

[57] CHOU R, QASEEM A, SNOW V, et al. Diagnosis and treatment of low back pain: a joint clinical practice guideline from the American College of Physicians and the American Pain Society [J]. Ann Intern Med, 2007, 147(7): 478-491.

[58] 梁繁荣，王华．针灸学 [M]. 北京：中国中医药出版社，2016:211.

Migraine is a common primary pain in the head with unilateral or bilateral throbbing pain, and some people also manifest nausea, vomiting, irritability and other symptoms. In the philosophy of traditional Chinese medicine, migraine is categorized as a "headache", and its pathogenesis is mainly related to "wind, phlegm, blood stasis, heat and deficiency", which interact and ultimately lead to blood stasis blocking the meridians and collaterals, and pain. The key to clinic diagnosis and treatment of migraine in traditional Chinese medicine lies in energizing the meridians and collaterals. Acupuncture can effectively reduce pain and improve the quality of life for patients; and it is easy to operate and has fewer adverse effects, so it has been widely used in clinical practice.

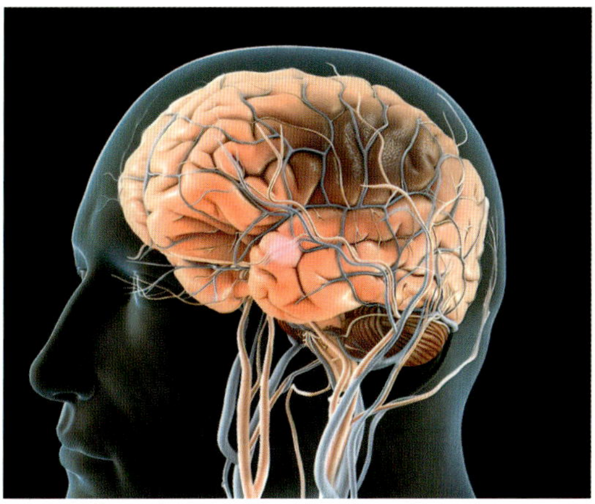

2）针灸治疗偏头痛临床疗效循证评价

2) Systematic evaluation of clinical effect of acupuncture on migraine

2016 年，一项纳入 22 个随机对照试验，共涉及 4985 名参与者的 Cochrane 系统评价显示[59]：现有证据表明，在头痛发作的对症治疗中加入针灸可减少头痛发作的频率。这与之前的研究结果相反，最新的证据还表明，针灸比假针灸有效果，但这种效果差异很小。现有的试验还表明，针灸的疗效可能至少与预防性药物治疗相似。对于愿意接受这种治疗的患者来说，针灸可被视为一种治疗选择（见表 8）。

[59] LINDE K, ALLAIS G, BRINKHAUS B, et al. Acupuncture for the prevention of episodic migraine [J]. Cochrane Database Syst Rev, 2016, 2016(6): CD001218.

In 2016, a Cochrane systematic review that included 22 RCTs involving a total of 4985 participants showed the available evidence suggested that adding acupuncture to symptomatic treatment of attacks reduced the frequency of headaches. Contrary to the previous findings, the updated evidence also suggested that there was an effect over control acupuncture, but this effect was small. The available trials also suggested that acupuncture might be at least similarly effective as treatment with prophylactic drugs. Acupuncture could be considered as a treatment option for patients willing to undergo this treatment (see table 8).

表 8　针灸治疗偏头痛临床疗效循证评价证据总结表

改善指标	对照类型	RCT 数量	试验组样本量	对照组样本量	SMD(95%CI)	GRADE 证据分级
头痛发作频率（治疗结束时）	针灸 vs 非针灸	4	1162	1037	SMD：−0.56 (−0.65 to −0.48)	中等
	针灸 vs 假针灸	12	952	694	SMD：−0.18 (−0.28 to −0.08)	中等
	针灸 vs 预防性药物	3	431	308	SMD：−0.25 (−0.39 to −0.10)	中等
随访期（12 个月）的头痛频率	针灸 vs 非针灸	1	152	132	SMD：−0.36 (−0.59 to −0.12)	低等
	针灸 vs 假针灸	10	896	638	SMD：−0.19 (−0.30 to −0.09)	中等
	针灸 vs 预防性药物	3	436	308	SMD：−0.13 (−0.28 to 0.01)	中等

Table 8　Summary of Evidence for the Effectiveness of Acupuncture in the Treatment of Chronic Nonspecific Migraine

Outcomes	Comparison	No. of Studies	No. of Patients		SMD (95%CI)	Certainty of the Evidence (GRADE)
			T	C		
Headache Frequency (After Treatment)	Acupuncture vs No Acupuncture	4	1162	1037	SMD: −0.56 (−0.65 to −0.48)	Moderate
	Acupuncture vs Sham Acupuncture	12	952	694	SMD: −0.18 (−0.28 to −0.08)	Moderate
	Acupuncture vs Prophylactic Drug Treatment	3	431	308	SMD: −0.25 (−0.39 to −0.10)	Moderate

continued table 8

Outcomes	Comparison	No. of Studies	No. of Patients		SMD (95%CI)	Certainty of the Evidence (GRADE)
			T	C		
Follow-up(12 Month) Headache Frequency	Acupuncture vs No Acupuncture	1	152	132	SMD: −0.36 (−0.59 to −0.12)	Low
	Acupuncture vs Sham Acupuncture	10	896	638	SMD: −0.19 (−0.30 to −0.09)	Moderate
	Acupuncture vs Prophylactic Drug Treatment	3	436	308	SMD: −0.13 (−0.28 to 0.01)	Moderate

3）针灸治疗偏头痛循证指南推荐

3) Clinical guideline recommendations for acupuncture in the treatment of migraine

全球范围内，共有 42 篇偏头痛防治指南提及了针灸治疗，其中 21 项对针灸有明确推荐意见（14 项推荐，7 项不推荐），21 项提及针灸但无明确推荐意见[60]。早在 1998 年，加拿大的 William E.M. Pryse-Phillips 教授等人编写的 *Guidelines for the Nonpharmacologic Management of Migraine in Clinical Practice. Canadian Headache Society*[61] 中，推荐捏脊、针灸等传统医学疗法治疗偏头痛，并将针灸评为 I 级证据，列为 B 级推荐。但在 2000 年后，美国神经病学学会等多个机构发布的偏头痛相关诊疗指南则由于高质量证据的相对缺乏，虽均提及针灸疗法，但未对针灸治疗偏头痛给出明确推荐。随着针灸治疗偏头痛的随机对照试验和系统评价逐年上升，特别是 2019 年和 2020 年两年，研究数量达到上涨高峰，针灸治疗偏头痛的有效性逐渐被世界认可。在 2021 年法国的 Demarquay 教授等人编写的 *Revised guidelines*

[60] 王小语，王京京，胡静，等．全球偏头痛防治指南中针灸推荐的现状分析 [C]// 世界针灸学会联合会，中国中医科学院，海南省卫生健康委员会．"中医针灸"申遗十周年特别活动暨世界针灸学会联合会 2020 国际针灸学术研讨会论文集 .2020:2.

[61] PRYSE-PHILLIPS WE, DODICK DW, EDMEADS JG, et al. Guidelines for the nonpharmacologic management of migraine in clinical practice. Canadian Headache Society [J]. CMAJ, 1998, 159(1): 47-54.

of the French Headache Society for the Diagnosis and Management of Migraine in Adults. Part 3: Non-pharmacological treatment [62] 中，对针灸治疗偏头痛的证据评分较高，并给予强力推荐。针灸治疗偏头痛临床指南推荐意见总结见图 9。

Globally, a total of 42 guidelines for the management of migraine mentioned acupuncture treatment, of which 21 had a clear recommendation for acupuncture (14 recommended, 7 did not recommend) and 21 mentioned acupuncture without a clear recommendation. As early as 1998, *Guidelines for the nonpharmacologic management of migraine in clinical practice*, written by Prof. William E.M. Pryse-Phillips and others in Canada, recommended for the first time chiropractic, acupuncture, and other traditional medical therapies for the treatment of migraine, and rated acupuncture as Class I evidence and classified it as a Class B recommendation. However, after 2000, migraine-related guidelines issued by the American Academy of Neurology and other organizations did not give a clear recommendation for the treatment of migraine with acupuncture due to the relative lack of high-quality evidence. As the number of RCTs and systematic evaluations of acupuncture for migraine has been rising year by year, especially in 2019 and 2020, the number of studies has reached a rising peak, and the effectiveness of acupuncture in treating migraine is gradually being recognized worldwide. In 2021, in the *Revised guidelines of the French headache society for the diagnosis and management of migraine in adults. Part 3: Non-pharmacological treatment* by the French Headache Society by Prof. Demarquay et al, the evidence for acupuncture for migraine was rated high and given a strong recommendation.Summary of clinical guideline recommendations for acupuncture in the treatment of migraine is shown in figure 9.

[62] DEMARQUAY G, MAWET J, GUÉGAN-MASSARDIER E, et al. Revised guidelines of the French headache society for the diagnosis and management of migraine in adults. Part 3: Non-pharmacological treatment [J]. Rev Neurol (Paris), 2021, 177(7): 753-759.

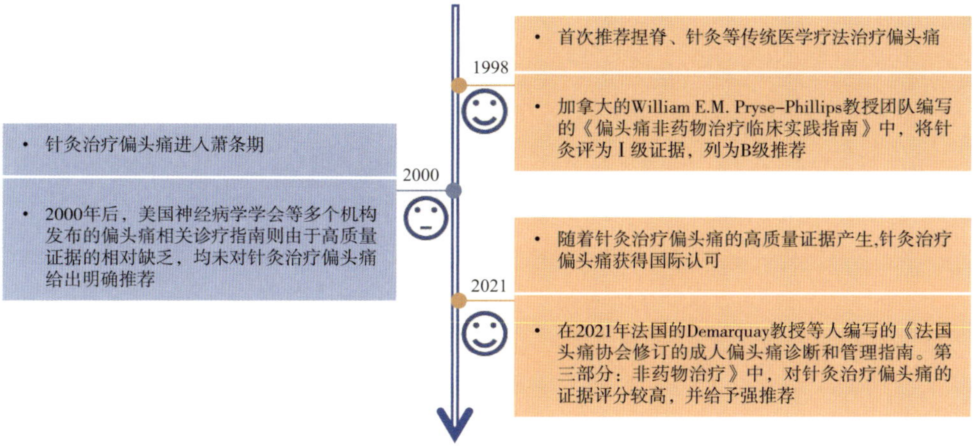

图 9　针灸治疗偏头痛临床指南推荐意见总结

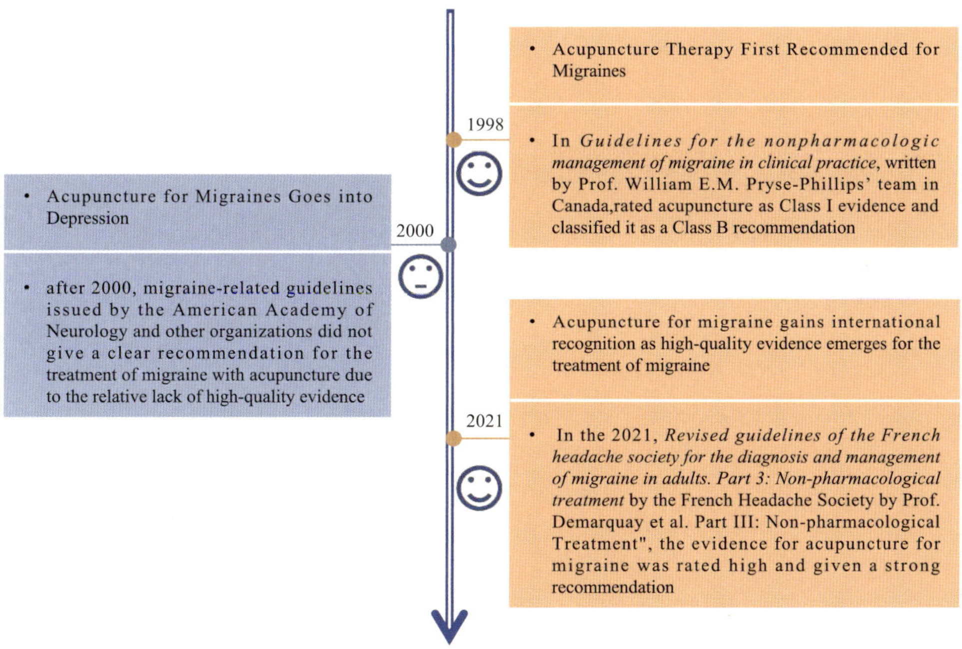

Figure 9　Summary of Clinical Guideline Recommendations for Acupuncture in the Treatment of Migraine

7. 轻度认知功能损害

7. Mild cognitive impairment (MCI)

1）针灸治疗轻度认知功能损害的机理

1) The mechanism of acupuncture in the treatment of stroke

轻度认知功能损害（MCI）被认为是健康老龄化过程中正常认知功能衰退与早期痴呆之间的过渡状态。它分为失忆亚型和非失忆亚型。MCI 是老年人最常见的疾病之一，会增加患痴呆症的风险。根据最新研究，MCI 患病率中国为 15.5%，希腊为 13.11%，南印度为 26.06%。此外，据报道，每年有 6% ～ 15% 的 MCI 患者会发展成阿尔茨海默病（AD），而每位阿尔茨海默病患者每年将花费 4 万美元用于治疗。MCI 向 AD 的高转化率给公共卫生带来了巨大的经济负担。因此，重视 MCI 的诊断和治疗至关重要。MCI 属于中医“痴呆”的范围，主要是由禀赋不足、痰浊阻窍、肝肾亏虚等引起。其病位在脑，与心、肝、脾、肾功能失调有关，病变多见虚实夹杂证。基本病机是髓海不足，神机失用[63]。针灸治疗轻度认知功能损害的作用机制主要是通过刺激特定的穴位，调节神经系统和内分泌系统，促进脑部血液循环，改善认知功能[64]。

Mild Cognitive Impairment (MCI) is considered to be a transitional period between normal cognitive decline and dementia in healthy aging. It is categorized into amnesic and non-amnesic subtypes. MCI is one of the most common disorders in elderly adults and increases the risk of developing dementia. According to recent studies, the prevalence of MCI among the elderly is 15.5% in China, 13.11% in Greece and 26.06% in South India. In addition, it has been reported that 6% ～ 15% of MCI patients develop Alzheimer's disease (AD) each year, at a cost of USD 40 000 per patient per annum. The high rate of progression from MCI to AD poses a significant economic burden to public health. Therefore, it is important to emphasize the diagnosis and treatment of MCI, which belongs to the scope of dementia in traditional Chinese medicine and is predominantly caused by insufficient vital energy, obstruction of the apertures by phlegm, deficiency of liver and kidney, etc. The disease is located in the brain and related to the dysfunction of the heart, liver, spleen and

---

[63] 梁繁荣，王华．针灸学 [M]. 北京：中国中医药出版社，2016:228.

[64] CHEN YX, LIANG N, LI XL, et al. Diagnosis and treatment for mild cognitive impairment: a systematic review of clinical practice guidelines and consensus statements [J]. Front Neurol, 2021, 12: 719849.

kidney, and mostly manifested as intermingled deficiency and excess. The basic pathogenesis is insufficiency of the brain and the disuse of the neurological mechanism. In treating mild cognitive impairment, acupuncture mainly works to stimulate specific acupoints, regulate the nervous system and endocrine system, promote blood circulation in the brain, and improve cognitive function.

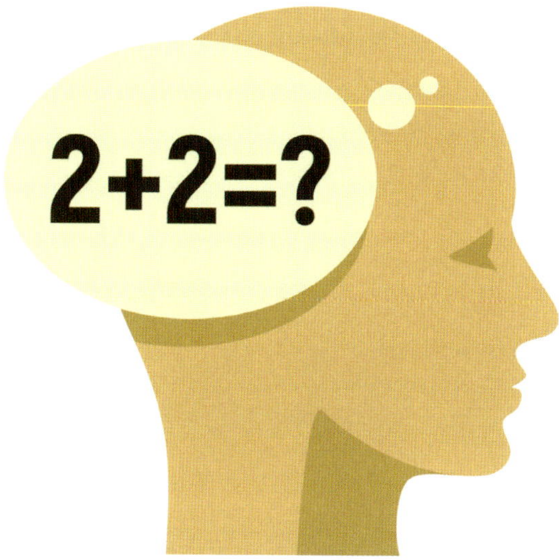

2）针灸治疗轻度认知功能损害临床疗效循证评价

2) Systematic evaluation of clinical effect of acupuncture on stroke

2023 年，一项共纳入 11 个随机对照试验，共涉及 602 名参与者的系统评价显示[65]：低确定性证据显示针灸显著提高了整体认知功能（OCF）[基于简易精神状态量表 (MMSE)、蒙特利尔认知评估量表 (MoCA) 测评]，在亚组分析中，与常规药物 (CM) 和假针灸 (SA) 相比，针灸显著增加了 MCI 患者的 OCF。试验序贯分析 (TSA) 的研究结果表明，针灸改善 MCI 患者 OCF 的证据是确凿的。同时，针灸与中药在改善记忆功能 (MF)（基于临床记忆量表（CMS）测评）、日常生活活动能力 (ADLs) 方面无统计学差异。TSA 显示，接受针灸治疗的 MCI 患者改善 MF 和 ADLs 的证据尚无定论。改善 MF 和 ADL 的证据从低到极低（见表 9）。

[65] YIN Z, LI Y, JIANG C, et al. Acupuncture for mild cognitive impairment: A systematic review with meta-analysis and trial sequential analysis [J]. Front Neurol, 2023, 13: 1091125.

In 2023, a systematic review that included 11 RCTs with a total of 602 patients. Low-certainty evidence showed that acupuncture significantly improved overall cognitive function (OCF) [Mini-Mental State Examination (MMSE); the Montreal Cognitive Assessment Scale (MoCA)]. In subgroup analyses, it was revealed that acupuncture significantly increased OCF in patients with MCI when compared to conventional medicine (CM) and sham acupuncture (SA). Trial sequential analysis's (TSA) findings indicated that the evidence of improving OCF with acupuncture for patients with MCI was conclusive. Meanwhile, there is no statistical difference in the improvement of memory function (MF) and activities of daily living (ADLs) between acupuncture and CM. TSA showed that the evidence of improving MF and ADLs for patients who had MCI and received acupuncture was inconclusive. The evidence of improving MF and ADL were ranked from low to critically low (see table 9).

表 9　针灸治疗轻度认知障碍临床疗效循证评价证据总结表

改善指标	对照类型	RC 数量	试验组样本量	对照组样本量	MD (95%CI)	GRADE 证据分级
MMSE	针灸 vs 常规药物	10	311	313	MD：1.22 (0.78 to 1.66)	低等
MoCA	针灸 vs 常规药物	7	169	170	MD：1.22 (0.47 to 1.97)	低等
CMS	针灸 vs 常规药物 *	2	29	33	MD：6.05 (−1.33 to 13.44)	低等
ADLs	针灸 vs 常规药物 *	2	60	60	MD：3.19 (−4.53 to 10.90)	极低等

注：针灸与常规药物之间没有统计学差异。

Table 9　Summary of Evidence for the Effectiveness of Acupuncture in the Treatment of Chronic Nonspecific MCI

Outcomes	Comparison	No. of Studies	No. of Patients		MD (95%CI)	Certainty of the Evidence (GRADE)
			T	C		
MMSE	Acupuncture vs Conventional Medicine	10	311	313	MD: 1.22 (0.78 to 1.66)	Low
MoCA	Acupuncture vs Conventional Medicine	7	169	170	MD: 1.22 (0.47 to 1.97)	Low
CMS	Acupuncture vs Conventional Medicine*	2	29	33	MD: 6.05 (−1.33 to 13.44)	Low
ADLs	Acupuncture vs Conventional Medicine*	2	60	60	MD: 3.19 (−4.53 to 10.90)	Very Low

Note: * There was no statistical difference between acupuncture and the conventional medicine.

3）针灸治疗轻度认知功能损害循证指南推荐

3) Clinical guideline recommendations for acupuncture in the treatment of MCI

在一项关于中医药治疗 MCI 指南的系统评价中提到，针灸治疗 MCI 效果良好[66]。2020 年，福建中医药大学团队基于当时已有的临床研究证据和专家经验，制定了针灸治疗轻度认知功能损害的专家共识[67]，专家共识详细描述了针灸治疗 MCI 的主穴，以及不同证型下的辨证配穴、针灸手法等，提供了借鉴价值，为针灸治疗 MCI 走向全球开启了新篇章。针灸治疗 MCI 临床指南推荐意见总结见图 10。

In a systematic evaluation of guidelines on was Chinese medicine for the treatment of MCI, it was mentioned that acupuncture was effective in the treatment of MCI. In 2020,the team from Fujian University of Traditional Chinese Medicine developed an expert consensus on acupuncture for mild cognitive impairment based on the clinical research evidence and expert experience available at that time. The guideline described in detail the main acupuncture points for acupuncture treatment of MCI, as well as the identification of matching points and acupuncture maneuvers under different types of evidence, which provided a reference value. The guideline described in detail the main points of acupuncture treatment for MCI, as well as the identification and matching points and acupuncture techniques for different types of evidence, which provided a reference value and opens a new chapter for the acupuncture treatment of MCI to the world.Summary of clinical guideline recommendations for acupuncture in the treatment of MCI is shown in figure 10.

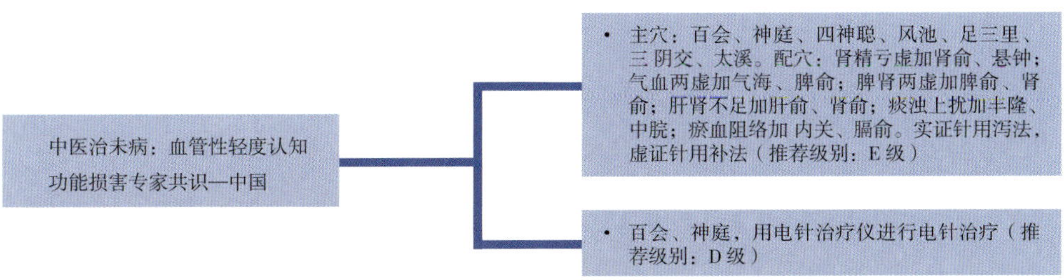

图 10　针灸治疗轻度认知功能损害临床指南推荐意见总结

[66] CHEN YX, LIANG N, LI XL, et al. Diagnosis and treatment for mild cognitive impairment: a systematic review of clinical practice guidelines and consensus statements [J]. Front Neurol, 2021, 12: 719849. doi:10.3389/fneur.2021.719849

[67] ZHOU XY, HUANG JS, Xie M, et al. Expert consensus for TCM preventive treatment of diseases: vascular mild cognitive impairment [J]. Chinese Journal of Information on Traditional Chinese Medicine, 2020, 27(3): 1-5.

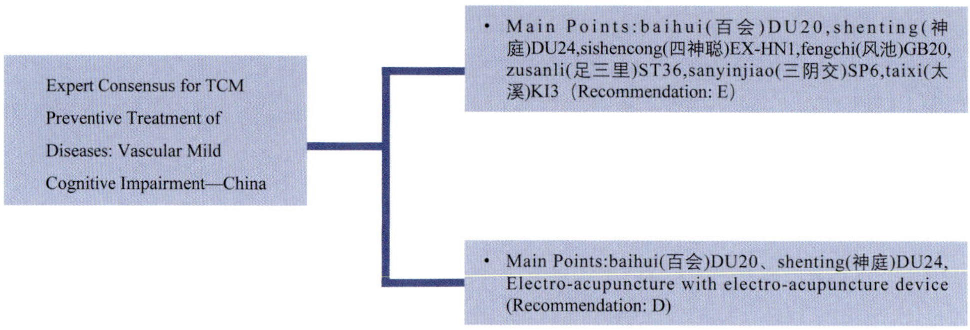

Figure 10 Summary of Clinical Guideline Recommendations for Acupuncture in the Treatment of MCI

8. 帕金森综合征

8. Parkinson's disease

1）针灸治疗帕金森综合征的机理

1)The mechanism of acupuncture in the treatment of Parkinson's disease

黑质纹状体通路内多巴胺能神经元的丧失是帕金森综合征（PD）最明确的病因之一。中医认为，帕金森综合征是本源不足、表面过剩所致。随着年龄的增长，脏腑功能逐渐下降，气血不足，出现了本源不足。在这种情况下，大脑不能得到营养，大脑骨髓越来越缺乏，导致病理变化[68]。根据中医理论，通过选择不同的穴位，针灸可以调节虚与实之间的平衡，以治疗疾病。机制研究[69]表明针灸通过促进内源性多巴胺的产生和增强多巴胺能神经元的存活，以及增强多巴胺的传递，使纹状体中的神经递质平衡正常化，这表明针灸可以用于帕金森综合征治疗。

[68] 陈松盛，李琛，杨颖，等. 补肾活血方对帕金森病大鼠多巴胺能神经元的保护作用及机制 [J]. 中国实验方剂学杂志，2014,20(21):175-179.

[69] FAN JQ, LU WJ, TAN WQ, et al. Acupuncture for arkinson's disease: From theory to practice [J]. Biomed Pharmacother, 2022, 149: 112907.

Loss of dopaminergic neurons within the nigrostriatal pathway is one of the clearest etiologic factors of Parkinson's disease. Traditional Chinese medicine theory holds that Parkinson's disease is caused by an insufficient bodily origin and excess surface. With the increase of age, the gradually declined internal organs in functions and the deficient qi and blood result in an insufficiency of the bodily origin. When that happens, the brain cannot be nourished and the bone marrow of the brain becomes increasingly deficient, leading to pathological changes. According to the theory of traditional Chinese medicine, acupuncture can regulate the balance between deficiencies to treat the disease by acupuncturing different acupuncture points. Studies have indicated that acupuncture normalizes the neurotransmitter balance in the striatum by promoting endogenous dopamine production and enhancing the survival of dopaminergic neurons, as well as enhancing dopamine transmission, which suggests that acupuncture can be helpful for Parkinson's disease treatment.

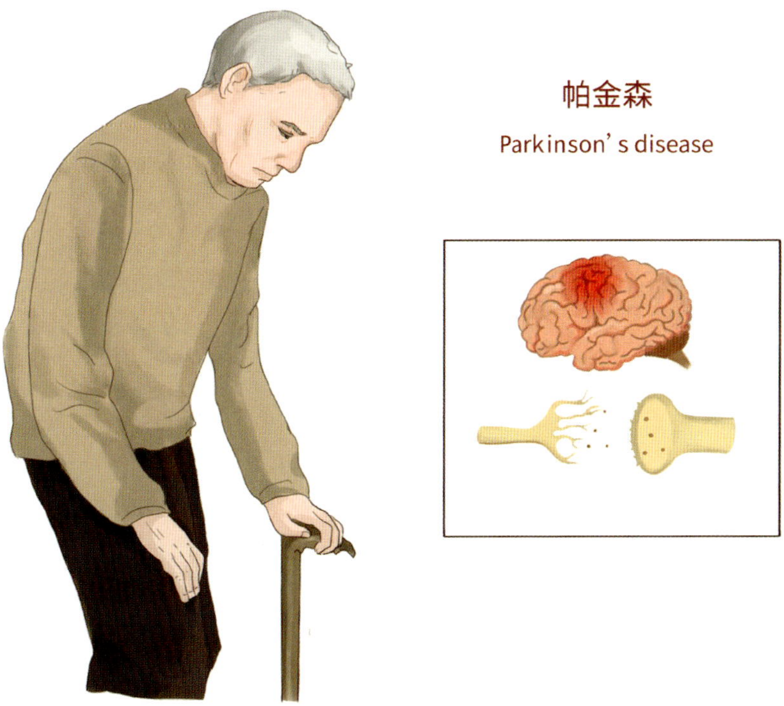

2）针灸治疗帕金森综合征临床疗效循证评价
2) Systematic evaluation of clinical effect of acupuncture on Parkinson's Disease

一项纳入 16 项随机对照试验，共涉及 462 名帕金森患者的系统评价显示[70]：针灸组在帕金森病评定量表 (UPDRS–III) 评分上优于对照组。定量 Meta 分析显示，针灸频率与运动症状 PD 患者 UPDRS–III 评分降低相关。在亚组分析中，一方面，当针灸次数不超过每周 3 次时，随着针灸次数的增加，UPDRS–III 评分的变化先降低后升高 (P = 0.000)。另一方面，当针灸每周超过 3 次时，针灸治疗的频率为 <60 次时，UPDRS–III 评分随针灸剂量的增加而增加，但剂量继续增加后，评分停止下降 (P =0.020)。两项定量随机对照试验的比较分析发现，每周针灸频率越高，UPDRS–III 评分改善越显著（见图 11，图 12）。

A systematic review included 16 studies involving 462 patients of Parkinson's disease (PD) showed that the acupuncture group had better effect on the Unified Parkinson's Disease Rating Scale Part III (UPDRS-III) scores than the control group. And the quantitative meta-analysis suggested that acupuncture dose was correlated with the reduction of UPDRS-III score in PD patients with motor symptoms. In subgroup analysis, on the one hand, when the frequency of acupuncture was no more than 3 times a week, with the increase of acupuncture session, the changes of UPDRS-III score decreased and then increased (*P=0.000*). On the other hand, when acupuncture for more than 3 times a week and the dose of acupuncture treatment was <60 times, the changes of UPDRS-III score increased with the increase of acupuncture dose, but the score stopped to decrease if the dose continued to increase (P = 0.020). The comparative analysis of two quantitative RCTs found that the score improvement was more significant at the higher weekly acupuncture frequency (see figure 11, figure 12).

[70] LEI S, FAN J, LIU X, et al. Qualitative and quantitative meta-analysis of acupuncture effects on the motor function of Parkinson's disease patients [J]. Front Neurosci, 2023, 17: 1125626.

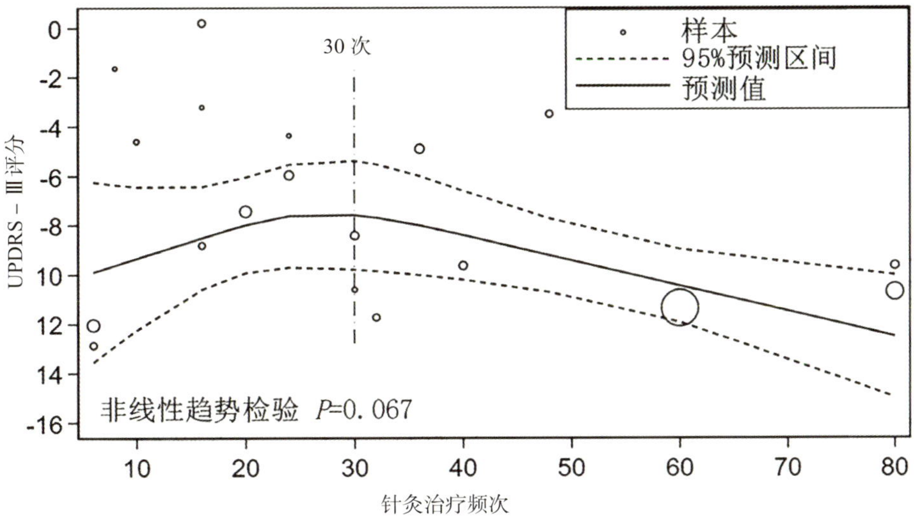

图 11　针灸治疗频率与 UPDRS—III 评分之间的非线性关系图

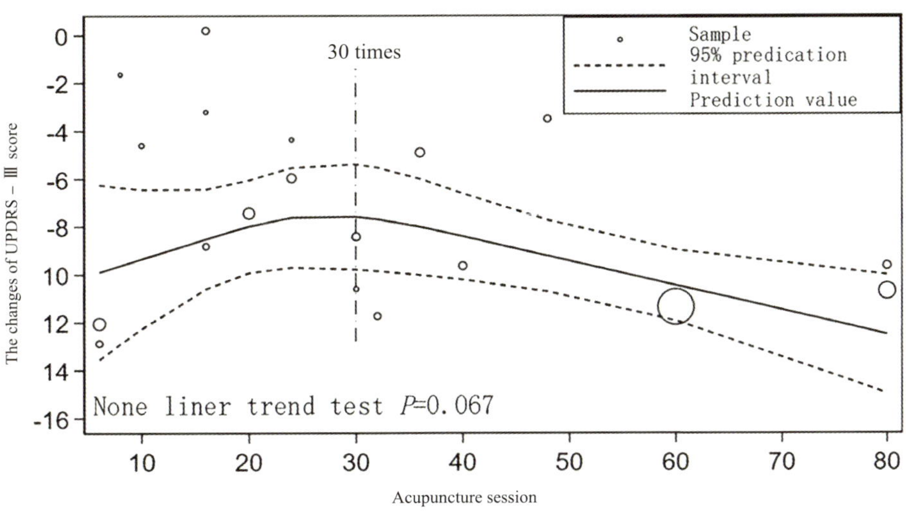

Figure11　Non-linear Relationship between Acupuncture Session and Changes of UPDRS-III Score

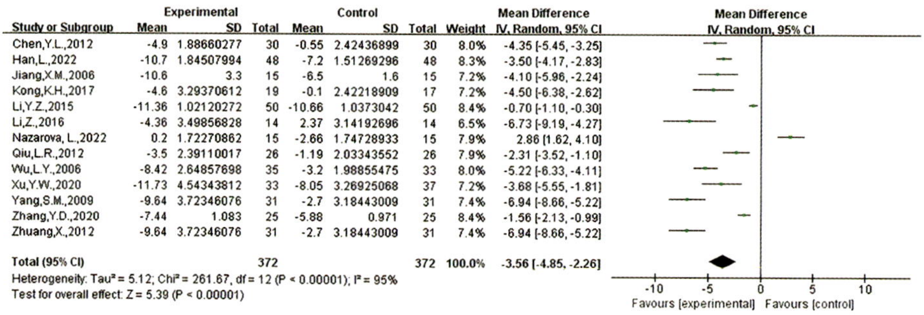

图 12　针灸组与对照组治疗前后关系的 Meta 分析

（Figure12　Meta-analysis of the Difference between Acupuncture Group and Control Group before and after Treatment）

3）针灸治疗帕金森综合征循证指南推荐

3) Clinical guideline recommendations for acupuncture in the treatment of Parkinson's disease

2012 年，加拿大神经科学联合会发布的帕金森指南 *Canadian Guidelines on Parkinson's Disease*[71] 中提及了针灸，但由于当时证据不足，未给出明确的建议。随后，2015 年，由中国上海曙光医院发布的 *A Practical Consensus Guideline for the Integrative Treatment of Parkinson's Disease* 中明确给出了针灸用于帕金森综合征的治疗，但此时的建议只是基于临床专家经验给出的，并没有基于系统评价证据 [72]。2018 年，韩国庆熙大学专家团队基于低可信度证据，给出了中等级别的建议 [73]：PD 患者应考虑同时使用针灸和抗帕金森药物治疗，并给出了具体的针灸治疗方案。针灸治疗帕金森综合征指南推荐意见总结见图 13。

Acupuncture for Parkinson's disease was first documented in *Canadian Guidelines on Parkinson's Disease* by the Canadian Neurological Sciences Federation in 2012. Subsequently,

[71] GRIMES D, GORDON J, SNELGROVE B, et al. Canadian guidelines on parkinson's disease [J]. Can J Neurol Sci, 2012, 39(4 Suppl 4): S1-S30.

[72] PAN WD, LIU J, CHEN XJ, et al. A practical consensus guideline for the integrative treatment of parkinson's disease in Shanghai, China [J]. Integrative Medicine International, 2015, 2 (1-2): 56–62.

[73] CHO KH, KIM TH, KWON S, et al. Complementary and alternative medicine for idiopathic parkinson's disease: an evidence-based clinical practice guideline[J]. Front Aging Neurosci. 2018, 10: 323.

2012

- 关于针灸、手法疗法、生物反馈或亚历山大技术在帕金森综合征治疗中的应用，目前尚缺乏足够的证据支持或反驳。AAN等级为U

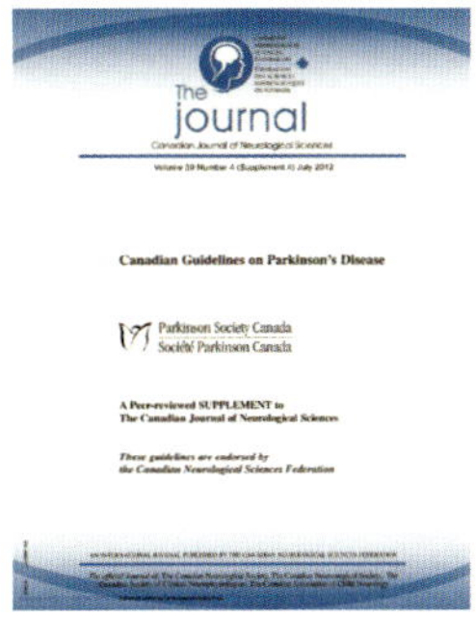

The journal

Canadian Guidelines on Parkinson's Disease

Parkinson Society Canada
Société Parkinson Canada

A Peer-reviewed SUPPLEMENT to
The Canadian Journal of Neurological Sciences

These guidelines are endorsed by
the Canadian Neurological Sciences Federation

2012年，加拿大神经科学联合会发布的《加拿大帕金森病指南》

2015

- 推荐意见：针灸和推拿经常被用作帕金森综合征患者的辅助治疗，可用于治疗运动和非运动症状；有时，这两种疗法被用于早发型帕金森综合征的初期管理，以延缓疾病进展。针灸师和推拿师可以根据中医理论选择穴位，这些穴位可以滋补肝肾的阴阳，或促进全身血液循环和/或消除血瘀

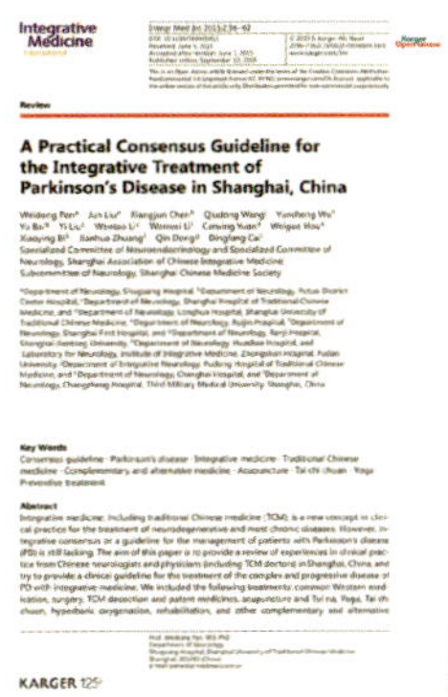

Integrative Medicine

Review

A Practical Consensus Guideline for the Integrative Treatment of Parkinson's Disease in Shanghai, China

KARGER

2015年，中国上海曙光医院发布了《帕金森病综合治疗实用共识指南》

2018

- 推荐意见：在特发性帕金森病（IPD）患者中，可以考虑同时使用针灸和抗帕金森药物疗法（推荐强度：B/证据水平：低）
- 针灸点如风池（GB20）、太冲（LR3）、阳陵泉（GB34）、合谷（LI4）、百会（GV20）、足三里（ST36）、曲泽（BL10）、天柱（BL40）、经典穴、太冲、涌泉、内关（PC6）可以考虑在针灸中使用

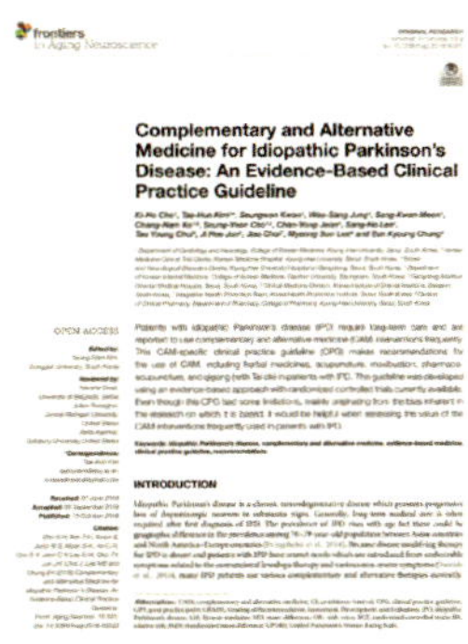

frontiers in Aging Neuroscience

Complementary and Alternative Medicine for Idiopathic Parkinson's Disease: An Evidence-Based Clinical Practice Guideline

OPEN ACCESS

INTRODUCTION

2018年，由韩国庆熙大学指南小组制定的《特发性帕金森病的补充和替代医学：基于证据的临床实践指南》

图 13　针灸治疗帕金森综合征指南推荐意见总结

2012

- There is insufficient evidence to support or refute the use of acupuncture, manual therapy, biofeedback or the Alexander technique in the treatment of PD. AAN Level U

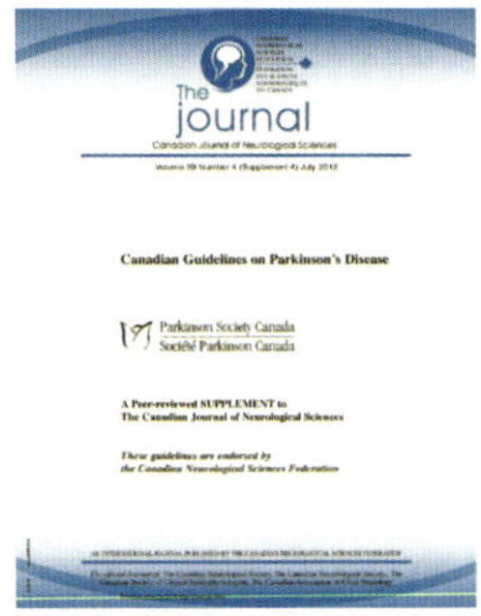

In 2012, *Canadian Guidelines on Parkinson's Disease* developed by the Canadian Neurological Sdences Federation

2015

- Statements: Acupuncture and"Tui na" (推拿, TCM massage) are often used as complementary treatments for PD patients with motor and non-motor symptoms; sometimes, the two therapies are used in early-onset PD as initial management to delay disease progression. Acupuncturists and massagers may choose acupoints according to TCM theory which may tonify the "yin" and "yang" of "Gan" and "Shen" or which may prompt the blood circulation of the body and/or remove blood stasis

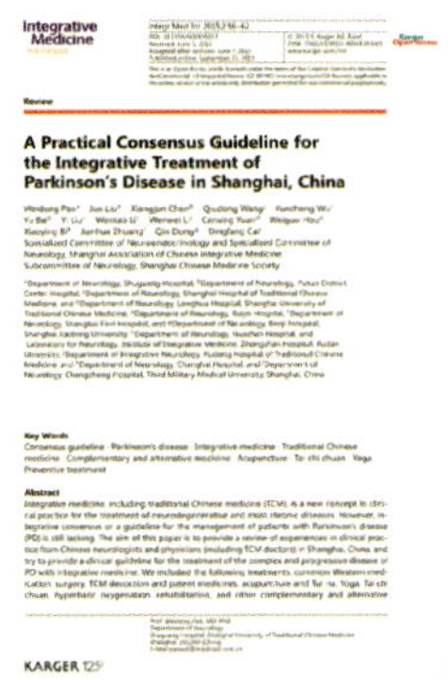

In 2015, *A Practical Consensus Guideline for the Integrative Treatment of Parkinson's Disease* released by Shanghai Shuguang Hospital China

2018

- Statements: Concomitant use of acupuncture and anti-parkinsonian drug therapy should be considered in patients with IPD (strength of recommendation: B/level of evidence: low)
- Acupuncture points such as GB20, LR3, GB34, LI4, GV20, KI39, LI11, GV16, BL10, BL40, GB6, GV1, and PC6 can be considered for use in acupuncture

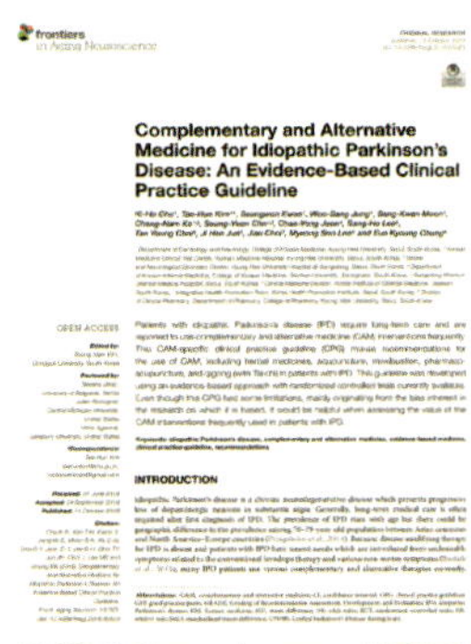

In 2018, *Complementary and Alternative Medicine for Idiopathic Parkinson's Disease: An Evidence-Based Clinical Practice Guideline* developed by guideline group from Kyung Hee University

Figure 13 Summary of Clinical Guideline Recommendations for Acupuncture in the Treatment of Parkinson's Disease

in 2015, *A Practical Consensus Guideline for the Integrative Treatment of Parkinson's Disease* released by Shanghai Shuguang Hospital in China clearly recommended acupuncture for the treatment of Parkinson's disease, but the recommendation was only based on clinical expert experience, and not based on systematic review. In 2018, guideline group from Kyung Hee University suggested that concomitant use of acupuncture and anti-parkinsonian drug therapy should be considered in patients with IPD, and provided the concrete acupuncture healing scheme. Summary of clinical guideline recommendations for acupuncture in the treatment of Parkinson's disease is shown in figure 13.

9. 坐骨神经痛

9. Sciatica

1）针灸治疗坐骨神经痛的机理

1) The mechanism of acupuncture in the treatment of sciatica

坐骨神经痛是一种主要表现为单侧腿部呈放射性疼痛，检查时伴或不伴有相关神经功能受损症状的疾病，常由腰椎间盘突出压迫腰骶神经根（L4 ～ S1）引起[74]。中医认为，坐骨神经痛归属于“腰腿痛”“坐臀风”“痹症”的范畴，认为本病多因受风寒湿邪，导致气血凝滞，经脉受阻，不通则痛[75]。针灸可以疏经理气、通络止痛、活血化瘀、濡养经脉，通过消除神经的炎性反应，抑制痛觉传导通路及神经递质的产生而产生治疗作用[76]。

Sciatica is a disease that mainly manifests as radiating pain in one side of the leg, with or without symptoms of related neurological impairment. It is often caused by lumbar disc herniation compressing the lumbosacral nerve root (L4~S1). Traditional Chinese medicine attributes sciatica to the category of “lumbar and leg pain” and “arthralgia syndrome”. It is believed that this disease is often caused by the invasion of external pathogenic wind, cold and

[74] JENSEN RK, KONGSTED A, KJAER P, et al. Diagnosis and treatment of sciatica [J]. BMJ, 2019, 367: l6273.

[75] 张浩琳，和岚，郭佳，等．早期针刺治疗腰椎间盘突出坐骨神经痛的临床疗效研究 [J]. 中国疼痛医学杂志，2020,26(2):146-149.

[76] 晋松，梁繁荣．坐骨神经痛的鉴别诊断与针灸循证治疗 [J]. 辽宁中医杂志，2011,38(10):1994-1995.

dampness, resulting in stagnation of qi and blood, blockage of meridians, and pain if blocked. Acupuncture can regulate the qi, clear and nurture the meridians and relieve pain, activate blood circulation, remove blood stasis, and produce therapeutic effects by eliminating the inflammatory reaction of the nerves and inhibiting the pain conduction pathway and neurotransmitter production.

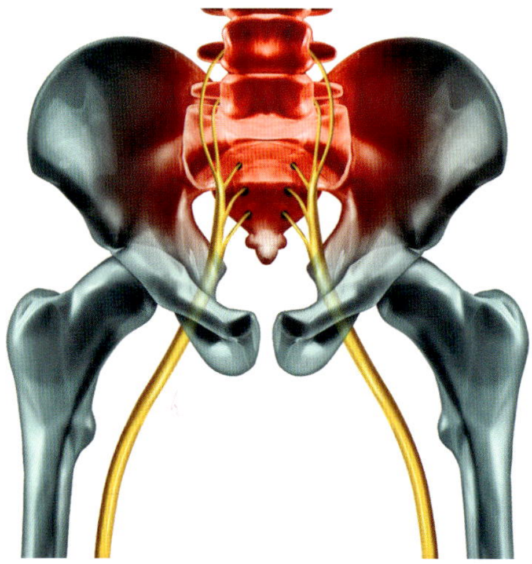

2）针灸治疗坐骨神经痛临床疗效循证评价

2) Systematic evaluation of clinical effect of acupuncture on sciatica

2023 年，一项纳入 30 个随机对照试验，共涉及 2662 名坐骨神经痛患者的系统评价显示：针灸在提高总有效率、降低视觉模拟量表（VAS）疼痛评分和提高疼痛阈值方面的临床疗效优于药物治疗。此外，在干预过程中出现的不良反应较少，这表明针灸是一种较安全的治疗方法[77]（见表 10）。

A total of 30 RCTs involving 2662 participants were included in the meta-analysis in 2023. The results showed that acupuncture was superior to that of medicine treatment in improving the total effective rate, reducing the Visual Analog Scale (VAS) pain score, and increasing pain threshold. In addition, few adverse events were reported during the

[77] ZHANG Z, HU T, HUANG P, et al. The efficacy and safety of acupuncture therapy for sciatica: a systematic review and meta-analysis of randomized controlled trails [J]. Front Neurosci, 2023, 17: 1097830.

intervention, which indicated that acupuncture was a safe treatment option (see table 10).

表 10　针灸治疗坐骨神经痛临床疗效循证评价证据总结表

改善指标	对照类型	纳入研究数量	试验组样本量	对照组样本量	SMD（或 RR）(95%CI)	GRADE 证据分级
总有效率[1]	针灸 vs 药物	26	1229	1203	RR: 1.25 (1.21 to 1.30)	中等
疼痛强度[2]	针灸 vs 药物	7	298	284	SMD: −1.77 (−1.89 to −1.66)	极低等
	针灸 vs 假针灸	2	60	59	SMD: −1.13 (−1.66 to −0.60)	低等
疼痛阈值	针灸 vs 药物	3	90	80	SMD: 2.07 (1.38 to 2.75)	极低等

注：SMD，标准平均差；RR，风险比；CI，置信区间。1，总有效率的计算方法是将治愈、明显好转和好转的患者人数除以患者总数。2，疼痛强度采用视觉模拟量表（VAS）测量，量表为 10 个等级（0 代表无痛，10 代表极度疼痛）。

Table 10　Summary of Evidence for the Effectiveness of Acupuncture in the Treatment of Sciatica

Outcomes	Comparison	No. of Studies	No. of Patients T	No. of Patients C	SMD (or RR) (95%CI)	Certainty of the Evidence (GRADE)
Total Effective Rate[1]	Acupuncture vs Medicine	26	1229	1203	RR: 1.25 (1.21 to 1.30)	Moderate
Pain Intensity[2]	Acupuncture vs Medicine	7	298	284	SMD: −1.77 (−1.89 to −1.66)	Very Low
	Acupuncture vs Sham Acupuncture	2	60	59	SMD: −1.13 (−1.66 to −0.60)	Low
Pain Threshold	Acupuncture vs Medicine	3	90	80	SMD: 2.07 (1.38 to 2.75)	Very Low

Note: SMD, standardized mean difference; RR,risk ratio; CI,confidence interval; T, treatment group; C,control group. 1, The total effective rate was calculated by dividing the number of cured, markedly improved, and improved patients by the number of total patients; 2, the pain intensity was measured by the Visual Analog Scale (VAS) with a 10-cm scale (0 cm represented no pain and 10 cm represented extreme pain).

3）针灸治疗坐骨神经痛循证指南推荐
3) Clinical guideline recommendations for acupuncture in the treatment of sciatica

2007 年，美国疼痛协会在指南中提及现有的证据不足以评估针灸治疗坐骨神经痛的有效性[78]。随着针灸治疗坐骨神经痛有效性证据的不断涌现，2021 年，北京中医药大学团队在改良德尔菲法的基础上，研制了针灸治疗坐骨神经痛的指南[79]，指南就坐骨神经痛针灸治疗的“剂量”（穴位选择、针灸频率和持续时间等）做出了如下推荐：

（1）由腰椎间盘突出引起的轻度、中度和严重坐骨神经痛，推荐使用针灸来改善临床症状（腰腿疼痛、肢体麻木、活动障碍、感觉异常、肌肉力量减退、生活质量和心理状态）。

（2）针灸治疗坐骨神经痛时，建议根据足太阳膀胱经和足少阳胆经进行经络辨证。建议的穴位包括腰夹脊 (EX–B2)、委中 (BL40)、环跳 (GB30)、阳陵泉 (GB34)、秩边（BL54) 和承山 (BL57)。

（3）推荐阿是穴的应用。

（4）推荐的阿是穴数量为 2 ～ 3 个。

（5）推荐针灸疗程持续 30 分钟，每周 3 次，治疗周期为 4 周。

针灸治疗坐骨神经痛临床指南推荐意见总结见图 14。

In 2007, the American Pain Society (APS) mentioned in its guideline that the available evidence was insufficient to assess the effectiveness of acupuncture for sciatica. As evidence of the effectiveness of acupuncture for sciatica continued to emerge, in 2021, the team from Beijing University of Chinese Medicine developed a guideline for the treatment of sciatica based on a modified Delphi method, which made recommendations on the “dose” of acupuncture for sciatica (selection of acupoints, frequency of acupuncture, and duration, etc.), as following:

(1) For the mild, moderate and severe sciatica caused by lumbar disc herniation, acupuncture is recommended to improve the clinical symptoms (lumbocrural pain, limb

---

[78] CHOU R, HUFFMAN LH, American Pain Society, et al. Nonpharmacologic therapies for acute and chronic low back pain: a review of the evidence for an American Pain Society/American College of Physicians clinical practice guideline [J]. Ann Intern Med, 2007, 147(7): 492–504.

[79] ZHANG N, WANG LQ, LI JL, et al. The management of sciatica by acupuncture: an expert consensus using the improved delphi survey [J]. J Pain Res, 2021, 14: 13–22.

numbness, activity disorder, sensory abnormality, muscle strength reduction, quality of life and mental state.

(2) The treatment of sciatica for acupuncture, it is suggested to meridians differentiation from the Bladder Meridian of Foot-Taiyang and Gallbladder Meridian of Foot-Shaoyang. It is suggested to pay attention to the application of points along meridians. The suggested acupoints are Yao jia ji (EX-B2), Wei zhong (BL40), Huan tiao (GB30), Yang ling quan (GB34), Zhi bian (BL54) and Cheng shan (BL57).

(3) It is suggested to pay attention to the application of Ashi point.

(4) The suggested number of Ashi is 2 ～ 3.

(5) The acupuncture stimulation is recommended to last for 30 min, the frequency is recommended to last for 3 sessions per week, and the period is recommended to last for 4 weeks.

Summary of clinical guideline recommendations for acupuncture in the treatment of sciatica is shown in figure 14.

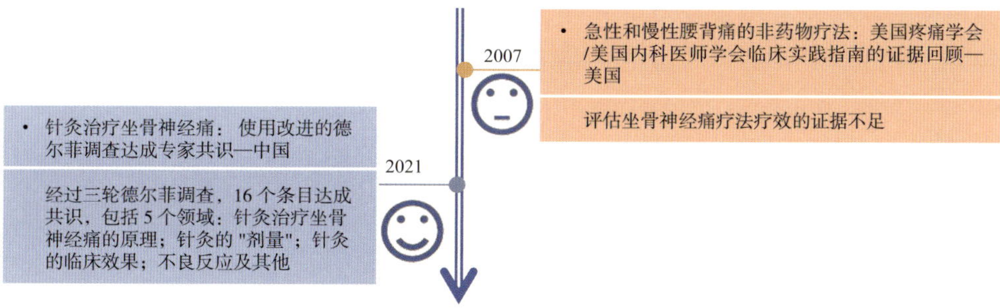

图 14　针灸治疗坐骨神经痛临床指南推荐意见总结

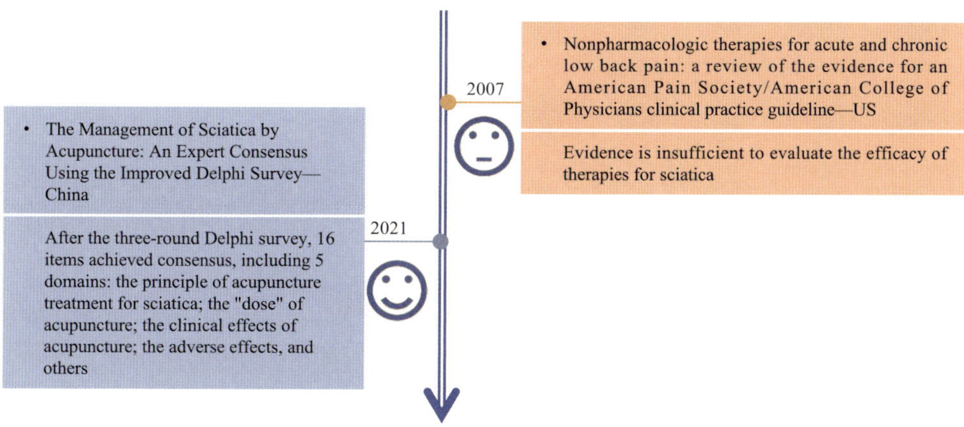

Figure14　Summary of Clinical Guideline Recommendations for Acupuncture in the Treatment of Sciatica

10. 脑卒中

10. Stroke

1）针灸治疗脑卒中的机理

1) The mechanism of acupuncture in the treatment of stroke

脑卒中，中医称为“中风”，以猝然昏仆、口舌歪斜、半身不遂、语言不利为主症，是最常见的致残和死亡原因。中医认为，中风主要为脏腑阴阳失调、气血逆乱，直冲犯脑，形成脑脉痹阻或者血溢脉外[80]。研究表明，针刺特定穴位可以促进神经细胞的生存和再生，通过神经递质的释放和神经元的连接，有助于康复过程。此外，针灸还能够减轻炎症反应，抑制炎性介质的释放，从而降低对脑组织的损害。血液循环的改善也是针灸治疗脑卒中的重要机制之一，有助于提供充足的氧和营养物质，促进受损脑区的修复。

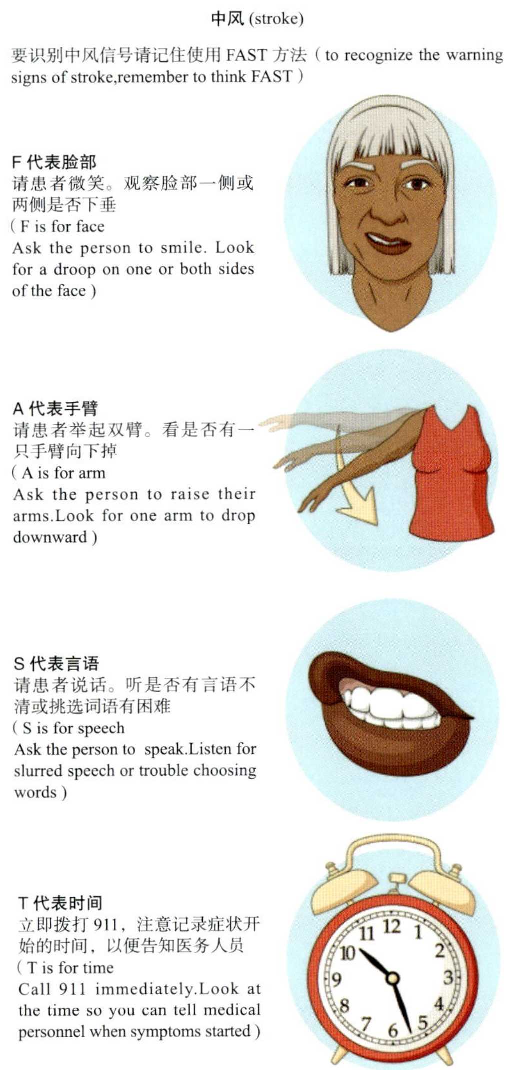

Known as “Zhong feng” in TCM, cerebral stroke is the most common cause of death and disability. The major symptoms of this disease are sudden fainting, crooked mouth and tongue, hemiplegia and slurred speech. TCM believes that stroke is mainly caused by the disharmony between yin and yang in

[80] 田烨楠，彭拥军 . 基于“从阴引阳，从阳引阴”探析针刺治疗中风思路 [J/OL]. 上海针灸杂志 ,1-6[2023-11-29]. https://doi.org/10.13460/j.issn.1005-0957.2023.13.0028.

the Zang and Fu as well as qi-blood disharmony, leading to a direct attack on the brain and resulting in paralysis of the cerebral veins or blood overflow. Studies suggest that acupuncture at specific points can promote the survival and regeneration of nerve cells, facilitating the recovery process through neurotransmitter release and neuronal connectivity. Additionally, acupuncture has the ability to reduce inflammatory responses by inhibiting the release of inflammatory mediators, thus lowering damage to brain tissues. Improved blood circulation is also a crucial mechanism in acupuncture treatment for stroke, providing sufficient oxygen and nutrients to promote repair in the damaged brain area.

2）针灸治疗脑卒中临床疗效循证评价

2) Systematic evaluation of clinical effect of acupuncture on stroke

2018 年，一项基于 33 项随机对照试验，共涉及 3946 名急性中风患者的 Cochrane 系统评价结果显示[81]：在使用任何对照比较的试验中，针灸组的参与者在随访结束时不太可能出现依赖或死亡，且更能改善神经功能缺陷，特别是运动功能。此外，2019 年，一项纳入了 28 项随机对照试验[82]，共涉及 1747 例患者的系统评价结果显示：针灸可以显著改善脑卒中后失语功能性沟通能力（见表 11）。

In 2018, a Cochrane systematic review included 33 RCTs with 3946 participants showed: across trials using any control comparison, participants in the acupuncture group were reported to be less likely to be dead or dependent at the end of follow-up and to have improved neurological deficits, especially for motor function. In 2019, another systematic review which included 28 RCTs involving 1747 patients demonstrated significant effects of acupuncture in improving functional communication measured by Chinese functional communication profile (CFCP) and communicative abilities of daily living (CADL) among patients with poststroke aphasia (see table 11).

---

[81] XU M, LI D, ZHANG S. Acupuncture for acute stroke [J]. Cochrane Database Syst Rev, 2018, 3(3): CD003317.

[82] ZHANG B, HAN Y, HUANG X, et al. Acupuncture is effective in improving functional communication in post-stroke aphasia: A systematic review and meta-analysis of randomized controlled trials [J]. Wien Klin Wochenschr, 2019, 131(9-10): 221-232.

表 11　针灸治疗脑卒中疗效评价的证据总结表

改善指标	对照类型	纳入研究数量	试验组样本量	对照组样本量	SDM（或 OR）（95%CI）	GRADE 证据分级
脑卒中后失语						
功能性性沟通能力[1]	手针 / 头针 / 传统与头针结合 + 康复 vs 康复	8	243	238	SMD：1.01 (0.81 to 1.2）	中等
急性脑卒中						
随访后患者的生存独立性[2]	针刺 vs 所有类型非针刺治疗	11	772	810	OR：0.61 (0.46 to 0.79)	极低等
随访 > 3 个月的患者的生存独立性		8	698	738	OR：0.67 (0.53 to 0.85)	极低等
治疗结束时整体神经功能缺损评分[3]		12	528	558	SMD：0.84 (0.36 to 1.32)	极低等
治疗结束时运动功能[4]		11	443	452	SMD：1.08（0.45 to 1.71）	极低等
随访后患者的生存独立性 *	针刺 vs 假针刺	4	124	138	OR：0.71 (0.43 to 1.18)	低等
随访 > 3 个月的患者的生存独立性 *		3	114	130	OR：0.67 (0.40 to 1.12)	低等
整体神经功能缺损评分 *		1	19	34	SMD：0.01 (−0.55 to 0.57)	低等
治疗结束时运动功能 *		3	101	101	SMD：−0.10 (−0.38 to 0.17)	低等

注： SMD，标准平均差；OR，比值比；CI，置信区间。1，功能性沟通能力时采用 Chinese functional communication profile (CFCP) 和 communicative abilities of daily living (CADL) 测量。2，独立性是指 BI 评分 ≤ 60（满分 100)，BI ≤ 70（满分 100)，或 BI ≤ 12（满分 20)。1 个研究采用了自定义的标准。3，整体神经功损失是采用 modified Edinburgh-Scandinavian Stroke Scale（9 个研究），NIHSS（2 个研究），and SSS（1 个研究）进行的测评。4，运动功能是采用 FuglMeyer Assessment（7 个研究），Motricity Index（1 个研究），motor function score（1 个研究），Rivermead Mobility Index（1 个研究）和 mobility index（1 个研究）进行测评。* 针刺与假针刺对比无统计学差异。

Table 11 Summary of Evidence for the Effectiveness of Acupuncture in the Treatment of Stroke

Outcomes	Comparison	No. of Studies	No. of Patients		SMD (or OR) (95%CI)	Certainty of the Evidence (GRADE)
			T	C		
Poststroke Aphasia						
Functional Communication[1]	MA/SA/TSA+RH vs RH	8	243	238	SMD: 1.01 (0.81 to 1.20)	Moderate
Acute stroke						
Death or Dependency[2] at End of Follow-up	Acupuncture vs All Control	11	772	810	OR: 0.61 (0.46 to 0.79)	Very Low
Death or Dependency at End of Follow-up (> 3 Months)		8	698	738	OR: 0.67 (0.53 to 0.85)	Very Low
Changes in Global Neurological Deficit Score[3] at End of Treatment Period		12	528	558	SMD: 0.84 (0.36 to 1.32)	Very Low
Motor Function Score[4] at End of Acupuncture Treatment Period		11	443	452	SMD: 1.08 (0.45 to 1.71)	Very Low
Death or Dependency at End of Follow-up[*]	Acupuncture vs Sham control	4	124	138	OR: 0.71 (0.43 to 1.18)	Low
Death or Dependency at End of Follow-up (> 3 Months)[*]		3	114	130	OR: 0.67 (0.40 to 1.12)	Low
Changes in Global Neurological Deficit Score at End of Treatment Period[*]	Acupuncture vs Sham Control	1	19	34	SMD: 0.01 (−0.55 to 0.57)	Low
Motor Function at End of Acupuncture Treatment Period[*]		3	101	101	SMD: −0.10 (−0.38 to 0.17)	Low

Note: SMD, standardized mean difference; OR, odds ratio; CI; Confidence interval; T,treatment group;C,control group.1, dependency was defined as BI ≤ 60 (of a potential total of 100), BI ≤ 70 (of a potential total of 100), or BI ≤ 12 (of a potential total of 20). One trial used the trialists' own definition. 2, Global neurological function was measured via modified Edinburgh-Scandinavian Stroke Scale in 9 trials, NIHSS in 2, and SSS in 1. 3, Motor function was measured via FuglMeyer Assessment in 7 trials, Motricity Index in 1, motor function score in 1, Rivermead Mobility Index in 1, and mobility index in 1. MA, manual acupuncture; SA, scalp acupuncture; TSA, traditional/scalp combined acupuncture; RH, rehabilitation. * There was no statistical difference between acupuncture and the sham control.

3）针灸治疗脑卒中循证指南推荐
3) Clinical guideline recommendations for acupuncture in the treatment of stoke

截至2021年，共48篇脑卒中指南中提及了84个针灸用于脑卒中治疗的建议[83]。其中42项对针灸用于卒中后遗症给出了积极建议，涉及14个症状领域：卒中康复、吞咽困难、肩痛、运动恢复、行走、平衡、痉挛、上肢障碍、卒中后疼痛、中枢性卒中后疼痛、认知障碍、抑郁、睡眠问题和急性卒中。针灸治疗脑卒中临床指南推荐意见总结见图15。

By 2021, a total of 48 stroke guidelines made 84 statements about acupuncture, 42 of which focus on the application of acupuncture in rehabilitation. Positive recommendations on the use of acupuncture were identified for 14 symptom: stroke rehabilitation, dysphagia, shoulder pain, motor recovery, walking, balance, spasticity, upper limb extremity impairment, post-stroke pain, central post stroke pain, cognitive disorder, depression, sleep problems,and acute apoplexy.Summary of clinical guideline recommendations for acupuncture in the treatment of stoke is shown in figure 15.

[83] BIRCH S, ROBINSON N. Acupuncture as a post-stroke treatment option: A narrative review of clinical guideline recommendations [J]. Phytomedicine, 2022, 104: 154297.

2005

- 英国国家医疗服务体系（NHS）中替代和补充医学的作用：对主流补充疗法对英国医疗保健的潜在贡献进行调查—英国

2006

- 渥太华专家组循证临床实践指南——卒中后康复—加拿大

2008

- 基于证据的卒中康复：欧洲卒中组织（ESO）2008年缺血性卒中和短暂性脑缺血发作管理指南的扩展指导文件—欧洲
- 加拿大卒中护理最佳实践建议（2008年更新）—加拿大

2009

- 德国神经康复学会指南——卒中后上肢运动治疗—德国
- 《神经病理性疼痛推荐指南手册》—中国香港
- 《卒中和短暂性脑缺血发作评估、调查、急救处理和二级预防指南》—新加坡
- 《针灸——辅助疗法，恶心呕吐和慢性疼痛病症医疗保险政策》—美国

2010

- SIGN 118. 卒中患者管理：康复、并发症预防和管理以及出院计划 国家临床指南—英国
- 卒中康复管理临床实践指南—美国
- 加拿大卒中护理最佳实践建议（2010年更新）—加拿大
- 中国急性缺血性卒中预防和治疗指南—中国
- 2010年临床指南—澳大利亚
- 新西兰卒中管理指南—新西兰

2011

- 《脑损伤康复——医疗技术评估主要报告》—丹麦
- 《中国卒中康复治疗指南（2011完整版）》—中国
- 《新加坡卫生部卒中和短暂性脑缺血发作临床实践指南》—新加坡

2012

- 国家卒中临床指南（第4版）—英国
- 卒中康复管理指南（简化版）—中国
- 神经性疼痛管理（第2版）—马来西亚

2013

- 指令6320.100 - 医疗、脊医学和持牌针灸—美国
- 加拿大卒中护理最佳实践建议：第四版—加拿大
- 疼痛性偏瘫性肩关节炎：卒中康复的循证评价—加拿大
- 卫生服务优先级：向州长和第77届俄勒冈州立法大会报告—美国
- 针灸（97810-97814）覆盖OHP/医疗补助，包括指南注释#92—美国

2014

- 美国心脏协会/美国卒中协会关于卒中的姑息治疗和临终关怀的声明—美国
- 中国今日卒中康复现状—中国
- 临床政策公告：针灸。编号：0135

2015

- S2e指南：卒中后运动康复（ReMoS）—德国
- 卒中和短暂性脑缺血发作——急性和长期管理—加拿大
- 加拿大卒中最佳实践建议：卒中后情绪、认知和疲劳实践指南，2015年更新—加拿大
- 针灸治疗卒中后痉挛性瘫痪的临床实践指南—韩国
- 针灸—美国

2016

- 国家卒中临床指南（第5版）—英国
- 卒中后吞咽困难：对未来试验的回顾和设计考虑—英国
- 成人卒中康复与恢复指南。来自美国心脏协会/美国卒中协会的医疗专业人士指南—美国
- 脑梗死和短暂性脑缺血发作—芬兰
- 加拿大卒中最佳实践建议：卒中康复实践指南，2015年更新—加拿大
- 基于质量的程序：卒中的临床手册（急性和亚急性）—加拿大

2017

- 脑梗死和脑出血指南数据库—荷兰
- 2017年临床指南—澳大利亚
- 临床政策公告：针灸。编号：0135—美国

2018

- 基于证据的卒中康复评估（第18版）—加拿大
- 中国卒中后抑郁临床实践指南—中国
- 指南与建议：新西兰卒中管理新临床指南2017年—新西兰
- 卒中后疼痛—英国

2019

- 临床指南：针灸服务（版本1.0.2019）针灸服务医疗必要性审查的临床指南—美国

2021

- 卒中后吞咽困难的诊断和治疗指南—欧洲

图 15　针灸治疗脑卒中临床指南推荐意见总结

2005

- The role of alternative and complementary medicine in the NHS: an investigation into the potential contribution of mainstream complementary therapies to healthcare in the UK—UK

2006

- Ottawa panel evidence-based clinical practice guidelines for post-stroke rehabilitation—Canada

2008

- Evidence-based stroke rehabilitation: an expanded guidance document from the European Stroke Organization (ESO) guidelines for management of ischaemic stroke and transient ischaemic attacks 2008—Europe
- Canadian best practice recommendations for stroke care (updated 2008)—Canada

2009

- Guideline of the German society for neurological rehabilitation motor therapies for the upper extremity for the treatment of stroke—Germany
- Handbook of neuropathic pain recommendation guidelines—Chinese Hong Kong
- Stroke and transient ischaemic attacks assessment, investigation, immediate management and secondary prevention——Singapore
- Acupuncture: adjunctive therapy, nausea and vomiting and chronic pain conditions medical coverage policy—US

2010

- SIGN 118. Management of patients with stroke: rehabilitation, prevention and management of complications, and discharge planning A national clinical guideline—UK
- Clinical practice guidelines for the management of stroke rehabilitation—US
- Canadian best practice recommendations for stroke care (Update 2010)—Canada
- Chinese guidelines on prevention and treatment for acute ischaemic stroke—China
- 2010 Clinical guidelines—Australia
- New Zealand guidelines for stroke Management—New Zealand

2011

- Brain injury rehabilitation: a medical technology assessment main report—Denmark
- Chinese guidelines on rehabilitation treatment for stroke (2011 full version)—China
- Singapore ministry of health clinical practice guidelines on stroke and transient ischemic attacks—Singapore

2012

- National clinical guideline for stroke （4th edition） —UK
- Guidelines on the management for stroke rehabilitation (simplify)—China
- Management of neuropathic pain （2nd edition） —Malaysia

2013

- BUMED instruction 6320.100 – Medical, chiropractic and licensed acupuncture—US BUMED
- Canadian best practice recommendations for stroke care: fourth edition—Canada
- Painful hemiplegic shoulder: evidence based review of stroke rehabilitation—Canada
- Prioritization of health services: a report to the governor and the 77th oregon legislative assembly—US
- Acupuncture (97810-97814) coverage ohp/medicaid, including guideline note #92—US

2014

- Palliative and end-of-life care in stroke: a statement for healthcare professionals from the American Heart Association/American Stroke Association—US
- Stroke rehabilitation in China today—China
- Clinical policy bulletin: acupuncture. number: 0135—US

2015

- S2e guideline rehabilitation of mobility after stroke (ReMoS)—Germany
- Stroke and transient ischemic attack – acute and long-term management—Canada
- Canadian stroke best practice recommendations: mood, cognition and fatigue following stroke practice guidelines, update 2015—Canada
- Clinical practice guideline on acupuncture for post-stroke spasticity—South Korea
- Acupuncture—US

2016

- National clinical guideline for stroke （5th edition） —UK
- Post-stroke dysphagia: A review and design considerations for future trials—UK
- Guidelines for Adult Stroke Rehabilitation and Recovery. A Guideline for Healthcare Professionals from the American Heart Association/ American Stroke Association—US
- Cerebral infarction and TIA—Finland
- Canadian stroke best practice recommendations: Stroke rehabilitation practice guidelines （update 2015） —Canada
- Quality-Based Procedures: Clinical Handbook for Stroke (Acute and Post-acute） —Canada

2017

- Richtlijnen database herseninfarct en hersenbloeding—Netherlands
- 2017 Clinical guidelines—Australia
- Clinical policy bulletin: acupuncture. number: 0135—US

2018

- Evidence based review of stroke rehabilitation (18th edition)—Canada
- Clinical practice guidelines for post-stroke depression in China—China
- Guidelines & Recommendations: New clinical guidelines for stroke management 2017—New Zealand
- Pain after stroke—UK

2019

- Clinical guidelines: acupuncture services. Version 1.0.2019. Clinical guidelines for medical necessity review of acupuncture services—US

2021

- Guideline for the diagnosis and treatment of post-stroke dysphagia—Europe

Figure15　Summary of Clinical Guideline Recommendations for Acupuncture in the Treatment of Stoke

三 针灸国际标准化

Chapter Three

International standardization of acupuncture

（一）针灸国际标准化发展历程
Part 1 The International Standardization Development of Acupuncture

针灸和草药一样，作为传统医学的一种重要治疗手段，在西太平洋地区应用已有 2500 多年的历史。因此，世界卫生组织西太平洋地区委员会分别于 1985 年和 1987 年正式通过了指导针灸和草药合理使用的决议 [84]。

为实现针灸标准化，1981 年，世界卫生组织西太平洋地区事务处 (WHO/WPRO) 组织成立了针灸命名标准化工作组 [85]。经过 10 年的努力，就关于针灸命名国际标准的提案取得共识。1991 年世界卫生组织总部出版发行了《国际针灸命名推荐标准》,WHO/WPRO 出版了《针灸命名标准》修订版 [86]。

作为经穴定位标准化的第一步，2003 年 10 月，WHO/WPRO 组织召开了关于制定 WHO 经穴定位标准的第一次非正式会议 [87]。2008 年世界卫生组织西太平洋地区委员会办公室颁布《世界卫生组织标准针灸经穴定位》(西太平洋地区)。

2014 年，国际标准化组织（ISO）正式出版了《ISO 17218:2014 中医药——一次性使用无菌针灸针》国际标准，这是 ISO 在世界传统医药领域发布的首个国际标准 [88]。

截至 2023 年 10 月，针灸已发布相关国际标准 14 项，其中中方主导 8 项。

Along with herbal medicine, acupuncture has been used for more than 2500 years as one

[84] WHO/WPRO. 世界卫生组织标准针灸经穴定位 (西太平洋地区)(中英文对照) [M]. 北京 : 人民卫生出版社 , 2010.

[85] 张瑞澄 , 郑元让 . 经络穴位命名朝向标准化 [J]. 广州中医学院学报 , 1986, (4): 8.

[86] 孙乃珺 , 张建斌 . 腧穴定位国标 1990 版与 2006 版的对比研究 [J]. 针灸临床杂志 ,2011,27(11):33-35.

[87] 秦秋 . WHO 第四次针灸经穴定位国际标准化会议在韩国举行 [N]. 中国中医药报 ,2005/05/09.

[88] 赵姝婷 , 钟燕梅 , 胡远樟 , 等 . 关于 ISO/TC 249 中医药国际标准可视化探析 (英文) [J]. Digital Chinese Medicine, 2022, 5 (2): 103-111.

of the main pillars of traditional medicine in the Western Pacific Region. Accordingly, the WHO Regional Committee for the Western Pacific adopted resolutions supporting the proper use of acupuncture and herbal medicine in 1985 and 1987 respectively.

With the aim of standardization in the field of acupuncture, the WHO Regional Office for the Western Pacific organized a Working Group for the Standardization of Acupuncture Nomenclature in 1981 and, after 10 years of effort, consensus was reached on the proposed standard international acupuncture nomenclature. In 1991, *A Proposed Standard International Acupuncture Nomenclature* was published by WHO Headquarters and a revised edition of *Standard Acupuncture Nomenclature* was published by the WHO Regional Office for the Western Pacific.

As an initial step in standardizing acupuncture point locations, the WHO Western Pacific Regional Office convened the first Informal Consultation on the Development of WHO Standard of Acupuncture Point Locations in October 2003. *The WHO Standard Acupuncture Point Locations in the Western Pacific Region* issued by the World Health Organization Regional Office for the Western Pacific, in 2008.

In 2014, the International Standardization Organization (ISO) officially published the "*ISO 17218:2014 Traditional Chinese Medicine — Sterile Acupuncture Needles for Single Use*" international standard, marking the first standard released by the ISO in the world of traditional medicine.

As of October 2023, 14 acupuncture-related international standards have been published, of which 8 were led by China.

（二）针灸国际标准（中方）

Part 2 Acupuncture international standards (China side)

1. 中医药——电针仪基础安全和性能的通用要求

1.Traditional Chinese medicine — General requirements for the basic safety and essential performance of electro-acupuncture stimulators

ISO 24571:2022[89]

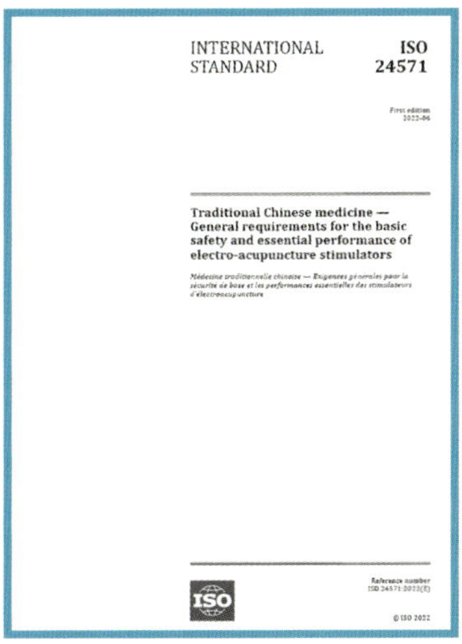

INTERNATIONAL STANDARD

ISO 24571

First edition 2022-06

Traditional Chinese medicine — General requirements for the basic safety and essential performance of electro-acupuncture stimulators

Médecine traditionnelle chinoise — Exigences générales pour la sécurité de base et les performances essentielles des stimulateurs d'électroacupuncture

Reference number ISO 24571:2022(E)

© ISO 2022

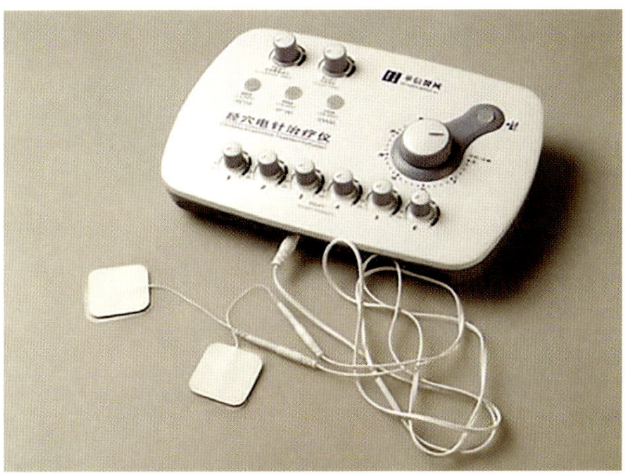

[89] ISO 24571:2022, Traditional Chinese medicine-General requirements for the basic safety and essential performance of electro-acupuncture stimulators.

标准内容

Standard content

1）提案国

1) Sponsors

中国

China

2）介绍

2) Introduction

本国际标准规定了电针仪的基本安全性和基本性能的一般要求。

为了方便医生和患者，电针通常被用来代替手针，这时手捻针就被施加于针柄上的电流刺激所代替，表现出同样的，甚至更强大的疗效。电刺激可以作用于肌肉、肌腱、结缔组织和神经等组织。电流很可能也会刺激到经络，但这方面的细致工作仍有待进行。由于电针的普遍使用，迫切需要建立一个国际标准，以保证其使用时的安全性和有效性。

This international standard specifies general requirements for the basic safety and essential performance of electroacupuncture (EA) stimulators.

For the convenience of the physicians and patients, the manual twisting of the needle has often been replaced by electrical stimulation applied on the needle shaft, and showed similar, even more favorable therapeutic effects. The stimulation is supposed to interact with the muscles, tendons, connective tissues and nerve fibers passing under the skin. Whether it would activate the hypothetical meridian or channels remains to be clarified. The popular use of electroacupuncture stimulator makes it urgent to set an international standard to guarantee its safe and effective use.

3）主要技术内容

3) Main technical elements

规范以下主要内容：①一般测试；②分类；③标签、标识和文件；④电安全防护；⑤机械安全防护；⑥要求；⑦电磁兼容性。

Standardizing the following technical index and elements: ①General requirements; ②Classification; ③Identification, marking and documents; ④Protection against electrical hazards; ⑤Protection against mechanical hazards; ⑥Requirement; ⑦Electromagnetic compatibility.

4）应用范围

4) Application range

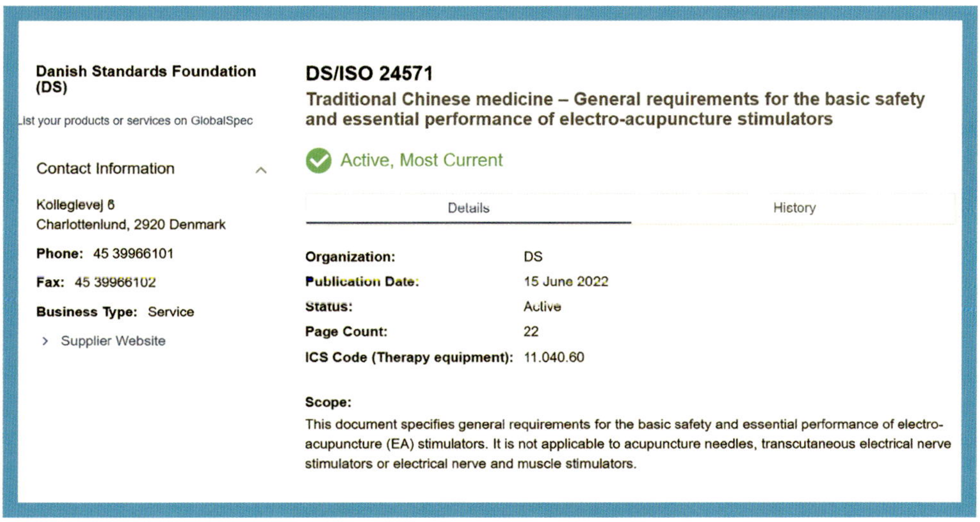
Danish Standards Foundation (DS)
List your products or services on GlobalSpec
Contact Information
Kollegievej 6
Charlottenlund, 2920 Denmark
Phone: 45 39966101
Fax: 45 39966102
Business Type: Service
Supplier Website
DS/ISO 24571
Traditional Chinese medicine – General requirements for the basic safety and essential performance of electro-acupuncture stimulators
Active, Most Current
Details
History
Organization: DS
Publication Date: 15 June 2022
Status: Active
Page Count: 22
ICS Code (Therapy equipment): 11.040.60
Scope:
This document specifies general requirements for the basic safety and essential performance of electro-acupuncture (EA) stimulators. It is not applicable to acupuncture needles, transcutaneous electrical nerve stimulators or electrical nerve and muscle stimulators.

丹麦

Denmark

丹麦：DS/ISO 24571 Traditional Chinese medicine — General requirements for the basic safety and essential performance of electro-acupuncture stimulators | GlobalSpec

2. 中医药——一次性使用无菌皮肤针——第一部分：叩击型

2.Traditional Chinese medicine — Dermal needles for single use — Part 1: Tapping-type

ISO 23958-1:2022 [90]

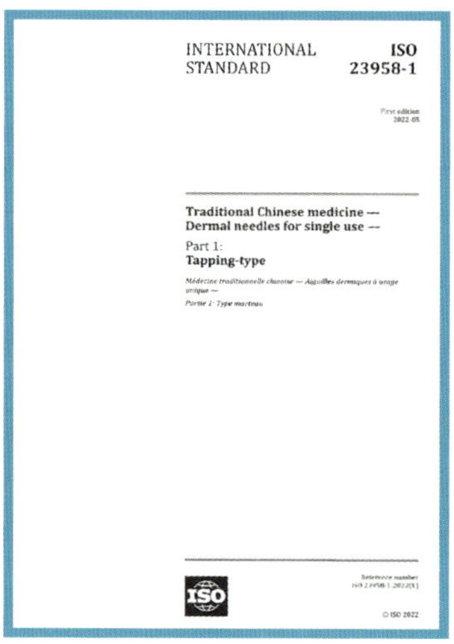
INTERNATIONAL STANDARD

ISO 23958-1

First edition
2022-05

Traditional Chinese medicine — Dermal needles for single use —

Part 1:
Tapping-type

Médecine traditionnelle chinoise — Aiguilles dermiques à usage unique —

Partie 1: Type marteau

Reference number
ISO 23958-1:2022(E)

© ISO 2022

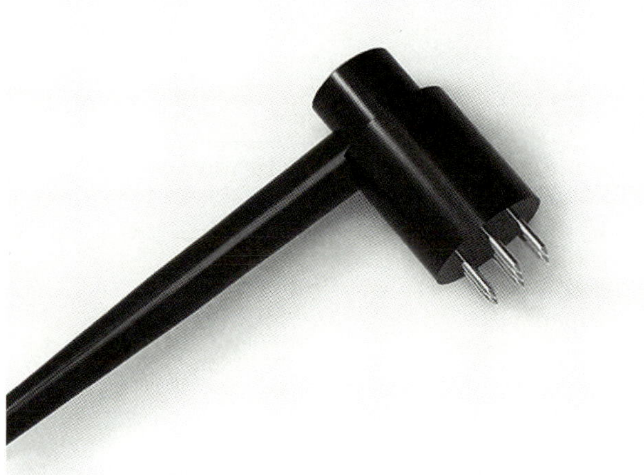

[90] ISO 23958-1:2022, Traditional Chinese medicine—Dermal needles for single use — Part 1: Tapping-type.

标准内容

Standard content

1）提案国

1) Sponsors

中国

China

2）介绍

2) Introduction

本国际标准规定了一次性使用的叩击型皮肤针的基本安全性和必要性能的特定要求。

运用皮肤针或结合其他疗法治疗临床各科疾病的临床经验常有报道，且涉及内、外、妇、儿、五官、皮肤、骨伤等各科病症。但在临床运用过程中，由于缺乏统一规范的针具，在进行皮肤针治疗时，易出现感染或其他不良反应。通过制定本标准，可保证皮肤针的有效性和安全性，便于推广皮肤针法，有利于皮肤针法的国内、国际交流，促进皮肤针法理论和技术的发展。

This international standard specifies the particular requirements for the basic safety and essential performance of tapping-type dermal needles for single use.

The clinical experiences of using a dermal needle or combining other therapies to treat various diseases are often reported. It is involved in internal medicine, surgery, gynecology, pediatrics, dermatology, orthopedics and other diseases. But in the process of clinical application, due to the lack of uniform standard of dermal needles, the infections and other side effects may be induced. By developing this standard, the effectiveness and safety of dermal needles can be ensured. It will be convenient to promote clinical use of dermal needles and beneficial to the domestic and international communication, which also promotes the development of the theory and technology of dermal needles.

3）主要技术内容

3) Main technical elements

规范以下主要内容：①材料、结构和规格；②针体要求；③针柄和针尖；④针尖的牢固性；⑤连接稳定性；⑥硬度要求；⑦耐腐蚀性；⑧产品包装；⑨运输和储存。

Standardizing the following technical index and elements: ①Materials, structure and dimensions; ②Needle body; ③Handle and tapping head; ④Firmness of needle tips; ⑤Fastness of connection; ⑥Hardness; ⑦Resistance to corrosion; ⑧Packaging; ⑨Transit and storage.

4）应用范围

4) Application range

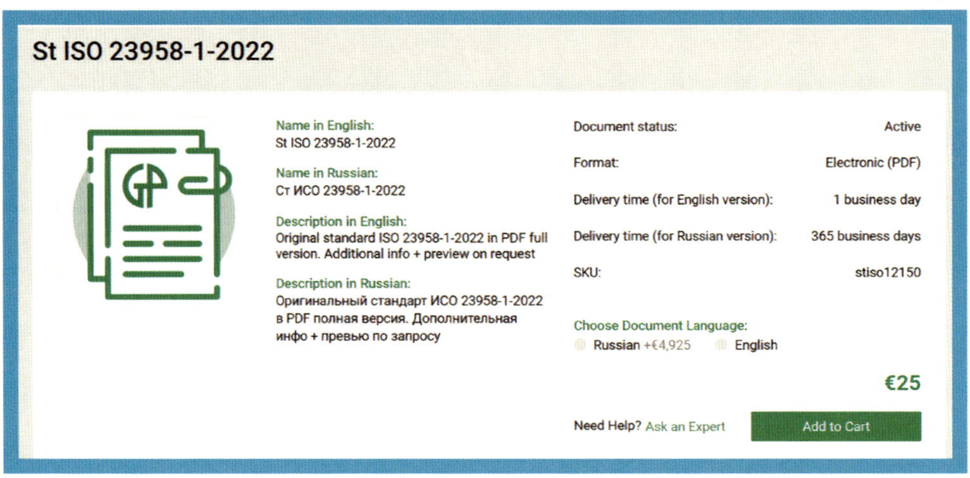
St ISO 23958-1-2022
Name in English:
St ISO 23958-1-2022
Name in Russian:
Ст ИСО 23958-1-2022
Description in English:
Original standard ISO 23958-1-2022 in PDF full version. Additional info + preview on request
Description in Russian:
Оригинальный стандарт ИСО 23958-1-2022 в PDF полная версия. Дополнительная инфо + превью по запросу
Document status: Active
Format: Electronic (PDF)
Delivery time (for English version): 1 business day
Delivery time (for Russian version): 365 business days
SKU: stiso12150
Choose Document Language:
Russian +€4,925
English
€25
Need Help? Ask an Expert
Add to Cart

日本

Japan

日本：St ISO 23958-1-2022 in English | Download PDF | GOSTPEREVOD.COM

3. 中医药——艾灸具通用要求

3. Traditional Chinese medicine — General requirements of moxibustion devices

ISO 18666:2021 [91]

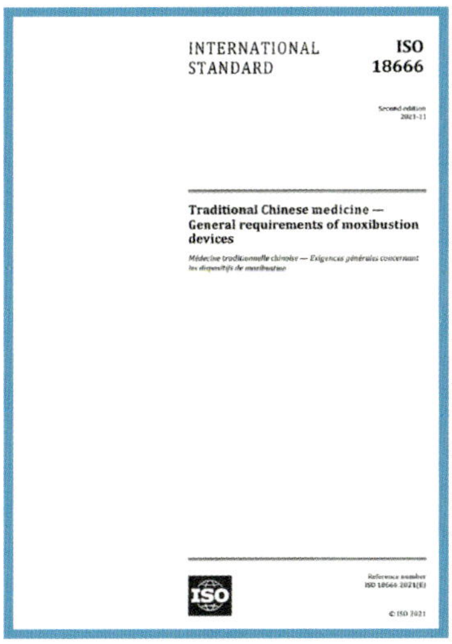

INTERNATIONAL STANDARD

ISO 18666

Second edition
2021-11

Traditional Chinese medicine — General requirements of moxibustion devices

Médecine traditionnelle chinoise — Exigences générales concernant les dispositifs de moxibustion

Reference number
ISO 18666:2021(E)

© ISO 2021

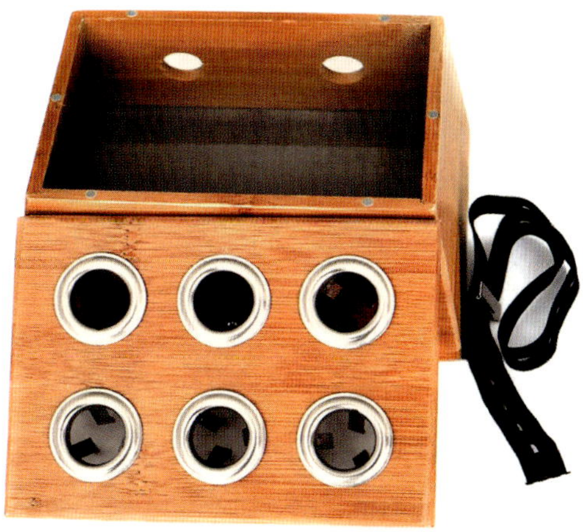

[91] ISO 18666:2021, Traditional Chinese medicine—General requirements of moxibustion devices.

标准内容
Standard content

1）提案国
1) Sponsors

中国

China

2）介绍
2) Introduction

本国际标准规定了艾灸器具的构造、材质、性能及安全要求，以及艾灸器具产品包装、标识、运输、储存和安全使用相关要求。本标准也规定了艾灸器具的性能检验方法，以及用于艾灸器具的艾绒和艾条的品质标准。

本国际标准适用于以燃烧艾绒为主要施灸方式，并在整个施灸过程中能安置或悬置于人体体表的艾灸器具。以电加热方式的艾灸器具以及手工施灸方式的艾绒和艾条不包括在本标准内。

This international standard specifies the structure, material, performance and safety requirements, as well as information concerning packing, labelling, transport, storage, and safe usage of moxibustion devices. This standard also includes the test methods for moxibustion devices and the general standard for moxa floss and moxa sticks used in moxibustion devices.

This international standard is applicable to all moxibustion devices that use moxa floss as the main combustion material and can remain on or over the body throughout the moxibustion process. Electro-moxibustion and moxa floss used in direct moxibustion are excluded in this standard.

3）主要技术内容

3) Main technical elements

规范以下主要内容：① 术语和定义；② 结构、材质和规格要求；③ 温度要求；④ 点燃方式；⑤ 施灸范围；⑥ 固定方式；⑦ 包装和标识；⑧ 运输和储藏；⑨ 使用要求。

Standardizing the following technical index and elements: ①Terms and definition; ②Structure, materials, and dimensions; ③Temperature; ④Ignition method; ⑤Area of moxibustion; ⑥Adhesion method; ⑦Packaging and labelling; ⑧Transport and storage; ⑨Information for use.

4）应用范围

4) Application range

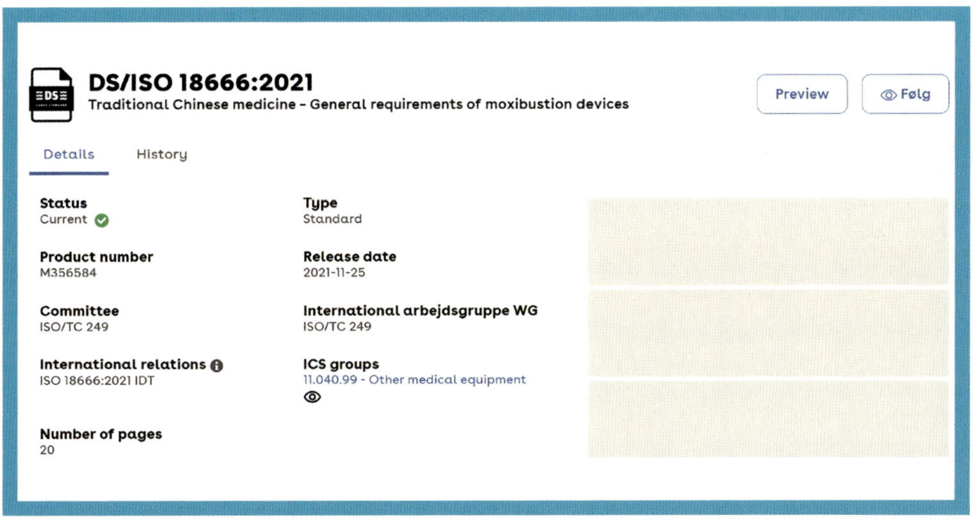

丹麦

Denmark

丹麦：DS/ISO 18666:2021 Webshop Dansk Standard

NEN-ISO 18666

Traditional Chinese medicine - General requirements of moxibustion devices

Active, Most Current

Details　　History　　References

Organization:	NEN
Publication Date:	1 November 2021
Status:	Active
Page Count:	22
ICS Code (Other medical equipment):	11.040.99

荷兰
Netherlands

荷兰: NEN-ISO 18666 Traditional Chinese medicine—General requirements of moxibustion devices | GlobalSpec

BS ISO 18666:2015　Current　Add to Watchlist

Traditional Chinese medicine. General requirements of moxibustion devices

Available format(s): Hardcopy, PDF

Language(s): English

Published date: 11-30-2015

Publisher: British Standards Institution

英国
United Kingdom

英国:BS ISO 18666:2015 Traditional Chinese medicine. General requirements (saiglobal.com)

4. 中医药——激光穴位设备

4.Traditional Chinese medicine—Laser acupoint devices

ISO 22466:2021 [92]

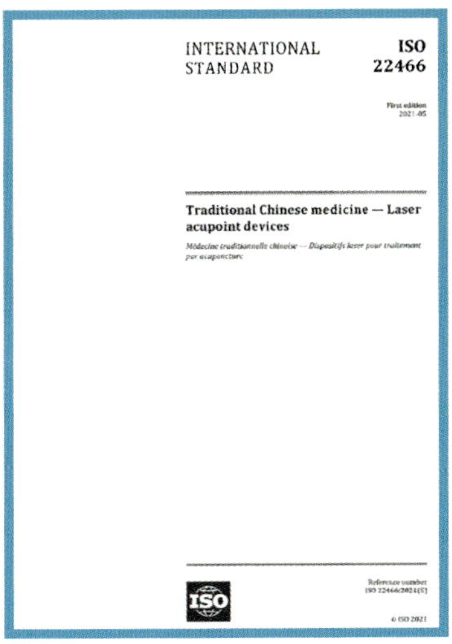

INTERNATIONAL STANDARD

ISO 22466

Traditional Chinese medicine — Laser acupoint devices

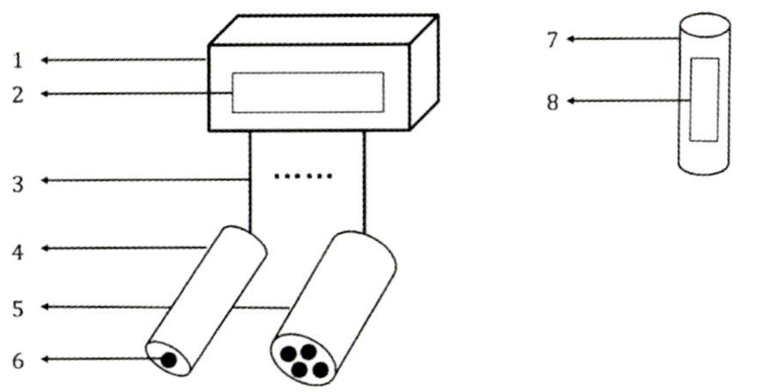

多探头－激光穴位设备
(multi-probe laser acupoint device)

单探头－激光穴位设备
(single-probe laser acupoint device)

1. 主机（mainframe）
2. 控制器（control unit）
3. 通路（channel）
4. 单束光辐射探测器（single beam radiation probe）
5. 簇束光辐射探测器（cluster beam radiation probe）
6. 激光束（laser beam）
7. 集成激光辐射探测器（integrated laser radiation probe）
8. 控制器（control unit）

[92] ISO 22466:2021, Traditional Chinese medicine—Laser acupoint devices.

标准内容

Standard content

1）提案国

1) Sponsors

中国

China

2）介绍

2) Introduction

本国际标准规定了激光穴位设备的要求和测试方法。不适用于二氧化碳型激光器。

This international standard specifies requirements and test methods for laser acupoint devices. This international standard is not applicable to carbon-dioxide-type lasers.

3）主要技术内容

3) Main technical elements

规范以下主要内容：①术语、定义；②分类；③波长；④光斑直径；⑤光强；⑥输出频率；⑦输出保护要求；⑧定时准确性；⑨材料的生物相容性；⑩附件要求；⑪使用说明书；⑫外部标记要求。

Standardizing the following technical index and elements: ①Terms and definitions; ②Classification; ③Wavelength; ④Beam diameter; ⑤Light intensity; ⑥Output frequency; ⑦Output protection; ⑧Time accuracy; ⑨Materials biocompatibility; ⑩Accessories; ⑪Instructions for use; ⑫Marking on the outside.

5. 中医药——一次性针灸埋线针针具

5. Traditional Chinese medicine — Thread-embedding acupuncture needle for single use

ISO 22236:2020 [93]

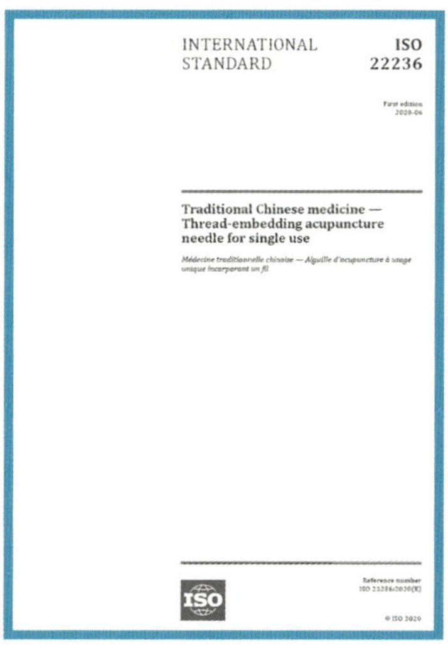

INTERNATIONAL STANDARD

ISO 22236

First edition 2020-06

Traditional Chinese medicine — Thread-embedding acupuncture needle for single use

Médecine traditionnelle chinoise — Aiguille d'acupuncture à usage unique incorporant un fil

Reference number ISO 22236:2020(E)

© ISO 2020

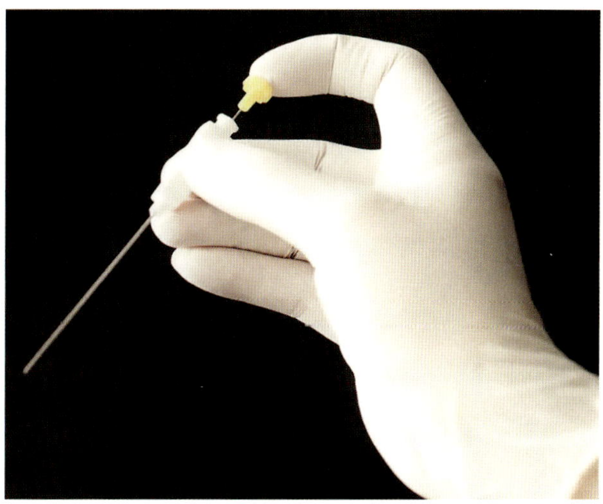

[93] ISO 22236:2020, Traditional Chinese medicine—Thread-embedding acupuncture needle for single use

标准内容

Standard content

1）提案国

1) Sponsors

中国

China

2）介绍

2) Introduction

本国际标准规定了一次性针灸埋线针的安全要求。适用于一次性针灸埋线针的针部分，不包括医用线。

近年来，现代针灸埋线疗法通过大量的临床研究论证，可有效治疗多种疾病。一次性针灸埋线针针具在世界多国及地区被广泛使用，包括美国、加拿大、俄罗斯、瑞士、伊朗、巴西、意大利、西班牙、新加坡、马来西亚。

This international standard specifies the safety requirements for the thread-embedding acupuncture needle. It is applicable to only the needle part of thread-embedding acupuncture needles and excludes medical thread.

In recent years, thread-embedding therapy has been demonstrated, by publication of numerous clinical research studies, to be effective in treating a variety of different conditions and diseases. The use of thread-embedding acupuncture needle has been widely accepted in many countries and areas, including America, Canada, Russia, Switzerland, Iran, Brazil, Italy, Spain, Singapore and Malaysia.

3）主要技术内容
3) Main technical elements

规范以下主要内容：①外观与尺寸；②针芯体和针腹体针部；③针芯体和针腹体尾部；④腹体针部；⑤化学性能；⑥生物性能；⑦刺穿力试验；⑧化学性能试验；⑨生物性能试验；⑩检验规则；⑪标志、标签；⑫使用说明书；⑬包装；⑭运输、贮存。

Standardizing the following technical index and elements: ①Appearance and size; ②Needle tube and needle core; ③Needle tube and needle core tail; ④Needle tube tip; ⑤Chemical properties; ⑥Biological properties; ⑦Pierce force test; ⑧Chemical properties test; ⑨Biological performance test; ⑩Inspection rules; ⑪Symbols and label; ⑫Instruction manual; ⑬Packaging; ⑭Transportation and storage.

4）应用范围
4) Application range

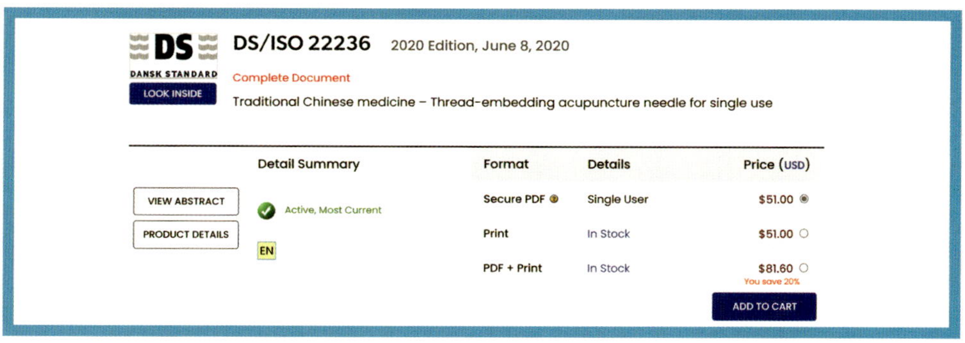

丹麦
Denmark

丹麦: DS/ISO 22236 Traditional Chinese medicine — Thread-embedding acupuncture needle for single use (ihs.com)

6. 中医药——一次性使用穴位磁疗贴

6. Traditional Chinese medicine — Acupoint magnetotherapy plaster for single use

ISO 22587:2023 [94]

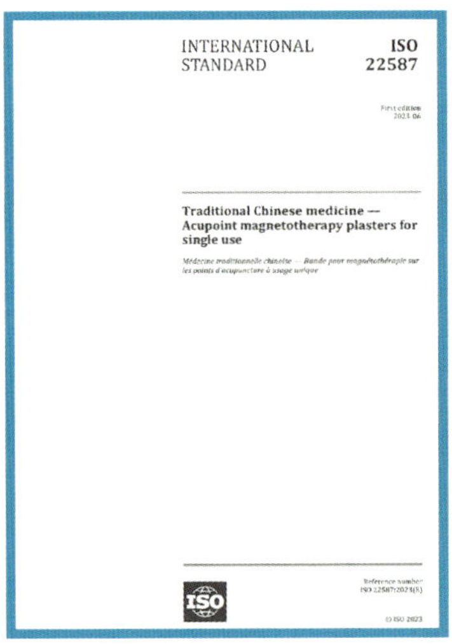
INTERNATIONAL STANDARD

ISO 22587

First edition 2023-06

Traditional Chinese medicine — Acupoint magnetotherapy plasters for single use

Médecine traditionnelle chinoise — Bande pour magnétothérapie sur les points d'acupuncture à usage unique

Reference number ISO 22587:2023(E)

© ISO 2023

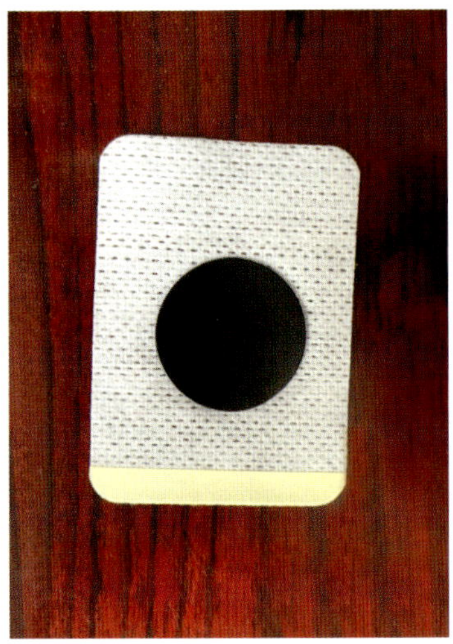

[94] ISO 22587:2023, Traditional Chinese medicine—Acupoint magnetotherapy plaster for single use.

标准内容

Standard content

1）提案国

1) Sponsors

中国

China

2）介绍

2) Introduction

本国际标准规定了穴位磁疗贴的基本安全和基本性能的要求。

在中国，穴位磁疗贴已经广泛使用。在中国已经获得中国食品药品监督管理局注册认可的品种有 100 余个。在国际市场上，世界其他国家如韩国、日本和加拿大也有着广泛的应用类似产品。该产品安全条款的缺失对患者存在一定的安全隐患。为了能够让穴位磁疗贴更好地在全球发展，有必要建立一个国际标准，对这类产品从安全性和有效性两方面进行规范。

This international standard specifies the requirements and test methods of single-use acupoint magnetotherapy plasters.

Acupoint Magnetotherapy Paster has been used extensively in China. There are more than 100 certifications of this kind of apparatus have been issued by CFDA. In the international market, other countries such as South Korea, Japan and Canada also have similar apparatus to be used extensively. It has some specific risks and performance of this kind of apparatus. To unify the understanding of the risk and performance, promote the market between different countries, there is need to establish an international standard.

3）主要技术内容
3) Main technical elements

规范以下主要内容：①材料与外观要求；②磁力；③磁场强度；④黏附强度；⑤外形尺寸；⑥包装和标签。

Standardizing the following technical index and elements: ①Material and appearance; ②Magnetic strength; ③Magnetic field strength; ④Adhesion strength; ⑤Geometric dimensions; ⑥Packaging and labelling.

4）应用范围
4) Application range

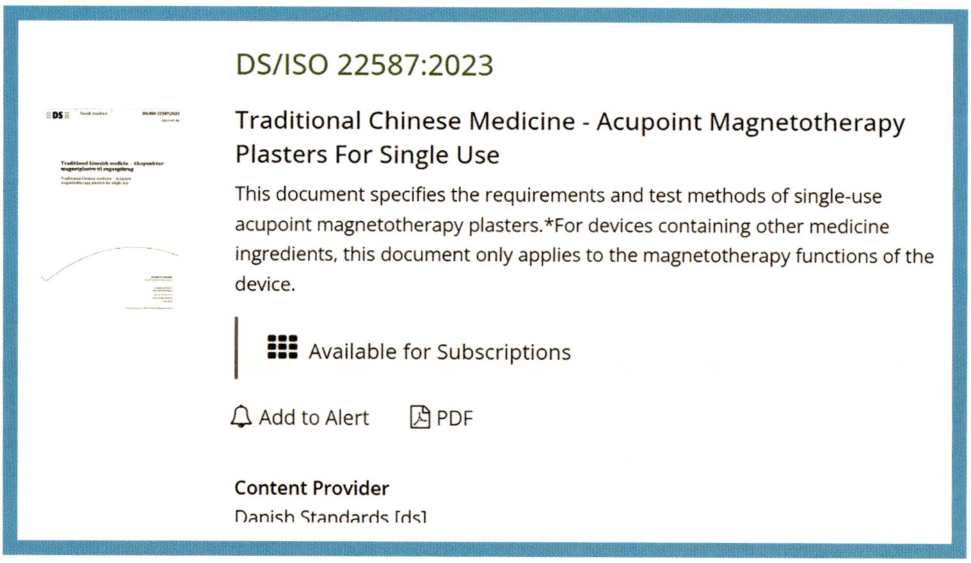
DS/ISO 22587:2023
Traditional Chinese Medicine - Acupoint Magnetotherapy Plasters For Single Use
This document specifies the requirements and test methods of single-use acupoint magnetotherapy plasters.*For devices containing other medicine ingredients, this document only applies to the magnetotherapy functions of the device.
Available for Subscriptions
Add to Alert
PDF
Content Provider
Danish Standards [ds]

丹麦
Denmark

丹麦：DS/ISO 22587 Traditional Chinese medicine—Acupoint magnetotherapy plasters for single use | GlobalSpec

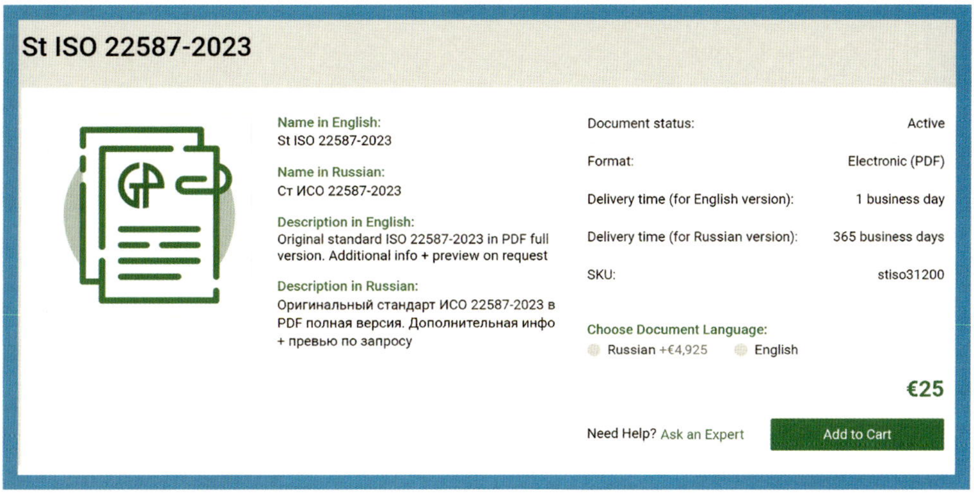

日本
Japan

日本: St ISO 22587-2023 in English | Download PDF | GOSTPEREVOD.COM

7. 中医药——红外灸疗仪

7.Traditional Chinese medicine — Infrared moxibustion-like instruments

ISO 20493:2018 [95]

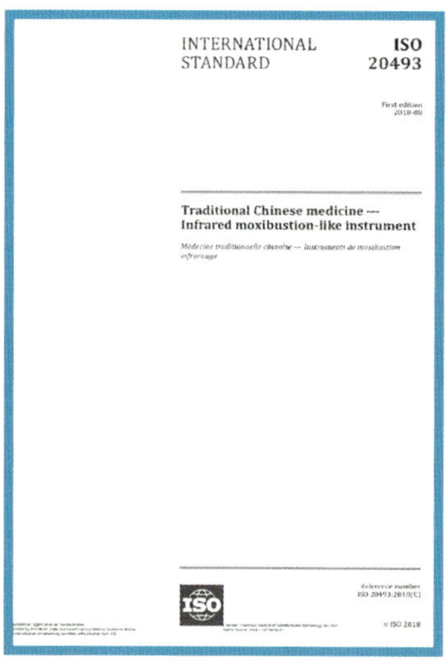

INTERNATIONAL STANDARD

ISO 20493

Traditional Chinese medicine — Infrared moxibustion-like instrument

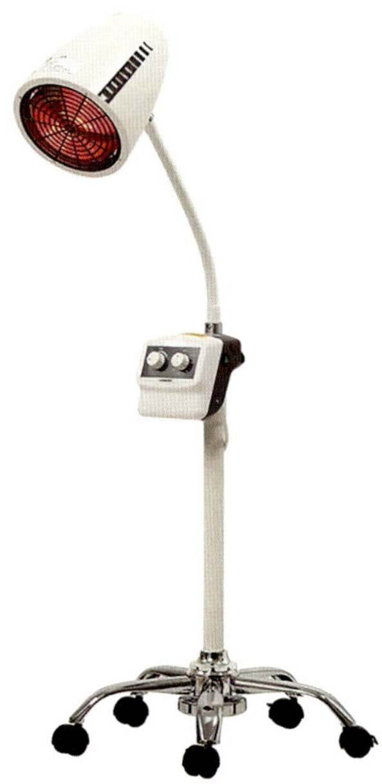

[95] ISO 20493:2018, Traditional Chinese medicine—Infrared moxibustion-like instruments.

标准内容

Standard content

1）提案国

1) Sponsors

中国

China

2）介绍

2) Introduction

本国际标准规定了红外灸疗仪作为医疗器械的要求。

TDP 是特定电磁波谱治疗仪，简称红外灸疗仪（商业名为“神灯”）。确定 TDP 治疗仪优势病种的相对应的波长，从而规范统一 TDP 治疗仪的波长范围；选择临床优势病种进行临床研究，从而确定针对所选优势病种的最佳治疗参数（照射的强度、照射的面积、照射的距离等治疗参数）；确定 TDP 治疗仪电器的安全范围，确定该仪器主要技术指标：波谱范围、功率密度、功率消耗、电源电压、工作条件等的国际标准。

This international standard specifies the requirements for infrared moxibustion-like instrument as a medical device.

TDP, a therapeutic device with specific electromagnetic spectrum, is referred to as infrared moxibustion-like instrument (commercially called “magic lamp”).To determine the corresponding wavelength of preferable diseases of TDP therapeutic device, thereby to standardize the wavelength range of the TDP therapeutic device; to select clinical preferable diseases for the clinical study so as to determine the optimal therapeutic parameters (intensity, area and distance of irradiation, and other therapeutic parameters); to determine the safety range of TDP therapeutic device; to determine the international standards of main technical indicators of the device, namely spectral range, power density, power consumption, power supply voltage, working conditions and so on.

3）主要技术内容
3) Main technical elements

规范其以下主要内容：①分类与命名；②波谱范围；③表面温度；④额定功率；⑤定时器范围；⑥使用寿命；⑦正常工作条件；⑧外观要求；⑨环境试验；⑩安全要求。

Standardizing the following technical index and elements: ①Classification and nomenclature; ②Spectral range; ③Surface temperature; ④Rated power; ⑤Timer range; ⑥Service life; ⑦Normal working conditions; ⑧Appearance requirements; ⑨Environmental tes; ⑩Safety requirements.

4）应用范围
4) Application range

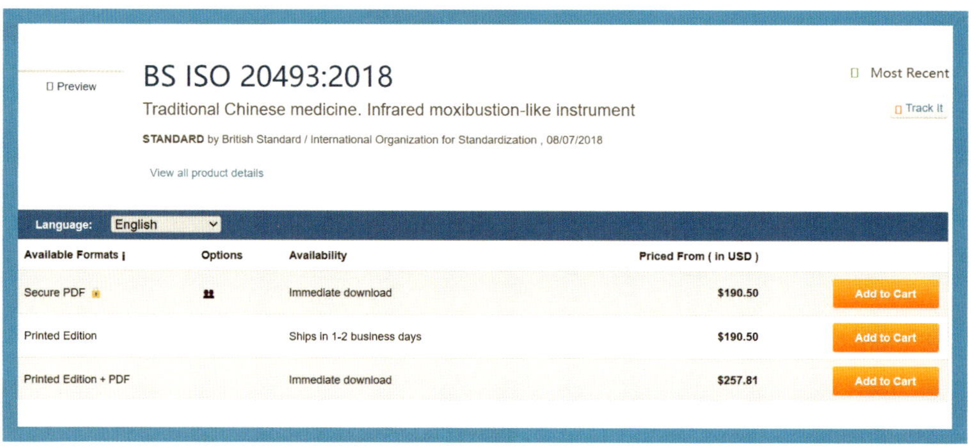

英国
United Kingdom

英国：BS ISO 20493:2018 Traditional Chinese medicine—Infrared moxibustion like instrument (British Standard) (ansi.org)

8. 中医药——一次性使用无菌针灸针

8.Traditional Chinese medicine—Sterile acupuncture needles for single use

ISO 17218:2014 [96]

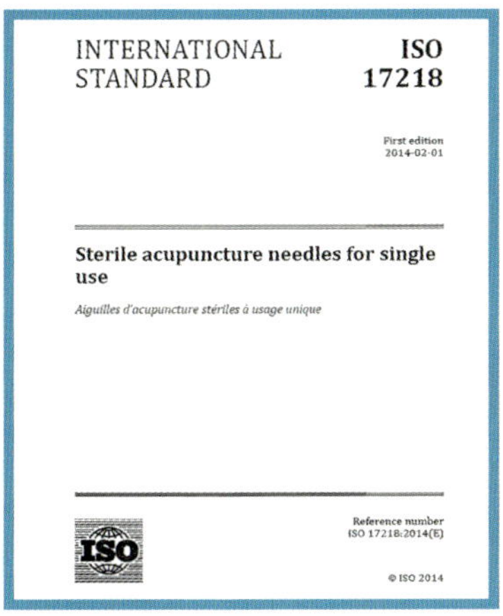
INTERNATIONAL STANDARD

ISO 17218

First edition 2014-02-01

Sterile acupuncture needles for single use

Aiguilles d'acupuncture stériles à usage unique

Reference number ISO 17218:2014(E)

© ISO 2014

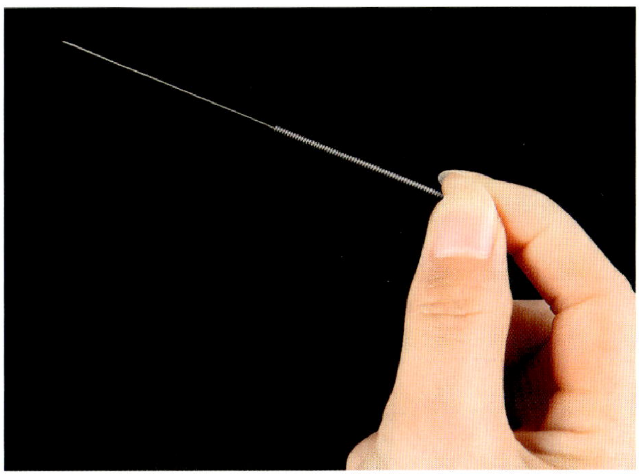

[96] ISO 17218:2014, Traditional Chinese medicine—Sterile acupuncture needles for single use.

标准内容

Standard content

1）提案国

1) Sponsors

中国

China

2）介绍

2) Introduction

本国际标准适用于针灸师用于针灸治疗的一次性无菌针灸针（毫针）。

This international standard applies to sterile acupuncture needles for single use (specialized for filiform needles) used by professional acupuncturists for acupuncture treatment.

3）主要技术内容

3) Main technical elements

规范其以下主要内容：①术语和名称；②结构和材质；③针尖形状；④直径及长度规格；⑤针体硬度与弹性要求；⑥针尖穿刺力的范围要求；⑦针体弹性的试验方法；⑧耐腐蚀性要求；⑨无菌要求；⑩包装、标签；⑪使用说明。

Standardizing the following technical index and elements: ①Terminology and nomenclature; ②Structure and material; ③The tip shapes; ④The diameter and length specifications; ⑤Hardness and flexibility; ⑥The range of puncturing force; ⑦The test methods of elasticity; ⑧Corrosion resistance; ⑨Sterility assurance; ⑩Packaging and labelling; ⑪Instructions for use.

4）应用范围
4) Application range

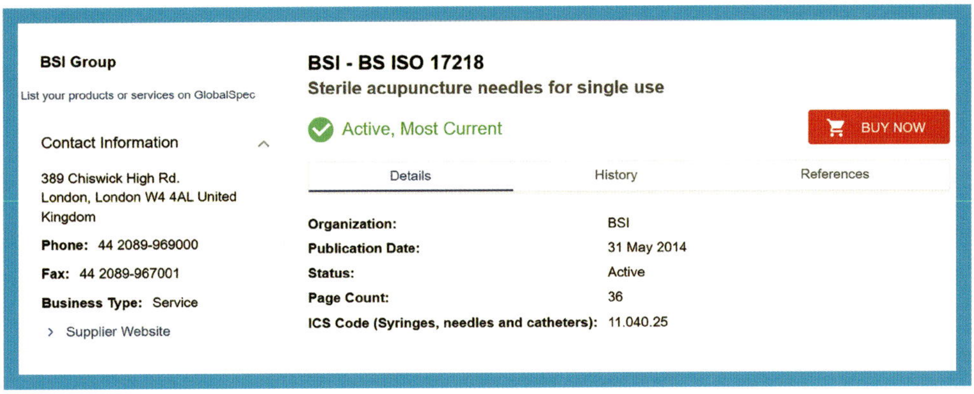

英国
United Kingdom

英国：BSI - BS ISO 17218 Sterile acupuncture needles for single use | GlobalSpec

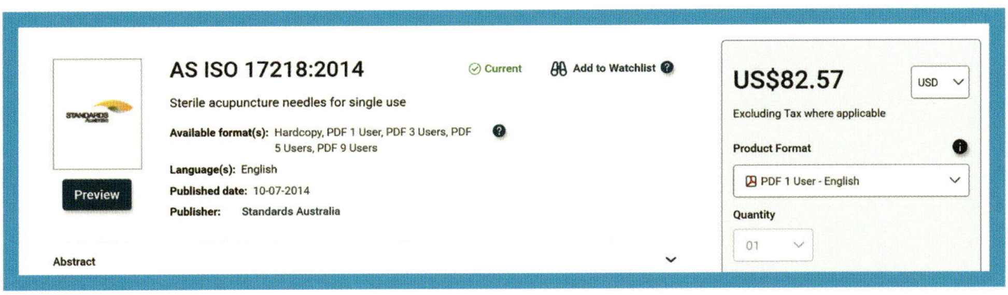

美国
United States

美国：AS ISO 17218:2014 | Sterile acupuncture needles for single use | (saiglobal.com)